Philosophy and Cognitive Science

ROYAL INSTITUTE OF PHILOSOPHY SUPPLEMENT: 34

EDITED BY

Christopher Hookway and Donald Peterson

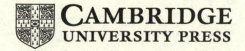

CAMBRIDGE UNIVERSITY PRESS

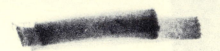

Published by the Press Syndicate of the University of Cambridge
The Pitt Building, Trumpington Street, Cambridge, CB2 1RP
40 West 20th Street, New York, NY 10011-4211, USA
10 Stamford Road, Oakleigh, Melbourne 3166, Australia

*A catalogue record for this book is available
from the British Library*

Library of Congress Cataloguing in Publication Data

Philosophy and cognitive science/edited by Christopher Hookway and
    Donald Peterson
        p. cm. —(Royal Institute of Philosophy supplement: 34)
    ISBN 0–521–45763–7
    1. Philosophy of mind. 2. Philosophy and cognitive science.
I. Hookway, Christopher. II. Peterson, Donald (Donald M.)
III. Series
BD418.3. P44 1993
128'.2—dc20   93–5719
                                                                          CIP

ISBN 0 521 45763 7 (paperback)

Origination by Michael Heath Ltd, Reigate, Surrey
Printed in Great Britain by the University Press, Cambridge

Contents

Preface

Possibly the most striking feature of research in the Philosophy of Mind during the last few decades has been the growing discussion of scientific investigations of mental phenomena: results from psychology and neuro-science are discussed; biological models of cognition have been judged relevant to a philosophical understanding of thought, perception, reasoning and other mental phenomena. This is surprising only against the background of the puritan approach to the mind characteristic of some other philosophical approaches. There have been those who saw no role for philosophy in moving beyond the analysis of psychological concepts to an interest in explanatory psychological theories. It is less so in the light of the history of philosophy. For example the empiricist tradition developed and used a distinctive (albeit flawed) theoretical model of cognition, the theory of ideas. If epistemologists are interested in the norms that govern reasoning and the search for knowledge, it is natural to expect them to benefit from our best knowledge of mental representation and the structure of inference.

The background to this growing interest in the sciences of mind is a more general breaking down of disciplinary boundaries. Those working in Artificial Intelligence have attempted to emulate various human cognitive achievements; psychologists have used computer simulations in formulating or testing hypotheses. Cognitive Science has emerged from this new and distinctively multi-disciplinary investigation of cognitive phenomena, of cognition and the mind. What unifies most of the studies under the umbrella of Cognitive Science is the use of computational, information processing models, techniques and concepts. The emergence of computers has produced new approaches to mental phenomena and new ways of thinking about the mind body problem: the earliest functionalist accounts of mind were presented through the assertion that the mind is a Turing machine. And computer simulations of complex cognitive activities provided ways of acquiring a new clarity about their structure and organization. Cognitive Science is now sufficiently unified and self-conscious that it has its own degree programmes, journals and academic conferences.

Philosophy engages with Cognitive Science in a number of ways. There are philosophers who react to it as yet another symptom of the philosophically confused idea that a 'science' of mind is either possible or desirable, or who insist that if it is possible it is of no philosophical importance. These views are not our concern here. Others are intrigued by the faltering attempts to forge a unified inter-disciplinary model of mind and address theoretical issues about the adequacy of computational models of mind and about the role of computer simulations in contributing to the understanding of mental phenomena. Still others seize on the growing repertoire of theories and concepts as ways of enriching their own thought about the mind, insisting that knowledge of psychological information and other material from Cognitive Science can contribute to our ability to make progress with traditional philosophical problems, and can make us aware of new philosophical problems about the mind and cognition. The hope is that interaction between those primarily involved in these different disciplines will be mutually beneficial.

The papers contained in this volume derive from a conference, sponsored by the Royal Institute of Philosophy, which was held at the University of Birmingham from 11 to 13 September 1992. Most have been revised, partly in the light of the discussion at what was a very rewarding, lively and enjoyable occasion. It is not our intention to provide a detailed introduction to them, but a few comments are in order. Some papers were concerned with particular mental phenomena, showing how knowledge of psychological research can help us to come to terms with the complexity of phenomena of traditional philosophical interests, while others are concerned with philosophical issues arising out of the attempt to develop cognitive models of psychological phenomena. Striking examples of the former include Michael Tye's discussion of blindsight and Andrew Woodfield's examination of some puzzling questions about the acquisition and growth of concepts. Stephen's Stich's development of his 'pragmatist' approach to epistemology is another example of how work in this area can be used to contribute to relatively traditional philosophical debates.

The papers concerned with the nature of cognitive science address a variety of issues: Aaron Sloman offers a general introduction to his distinctive view of the role and nature of work in artificial intelligence and Antony Galton offers a computer scientist's perspective on some foundational issues. It is no surprise that an issue of great theoretical importance within Cognitive Science—but also of considerable philosophical interest—receives most attention. This is the controversy between two general approaches to the study of cognitive phenomena, the debate between 'classical cognitivism' and connectionism. Classical cognitivism takes its inspiration from work in artificial intelligence, and sees the mind as a symbol processing system in which explicit symbolic data are manipulated by the application of rules. The connectionist view, on the other hand, takes its inspiration from work with artificial 'neural networks', and sees knowledge as essentially involving patterns of 'activation' and 'weighting' over networks of neurons. It is an open question how far these views are incompatible; and there has been extensive discussion of the theoretical underpinnings and importance of the new connectionist approaches. Several of the papers in this volume, contributed by philosophers and others involved in cognitive science, push these debates further; and the contribution of Stephen Mills discusses the intriguing relations between connectionist approaches to cognitive modelling and the view of the mind found in the work of Ludwig Wittgenstein.

Christopher Hookway
Department of Philosophy, University of Birmingham

Donald Peterson
Department of Computer Science, University of Birmingham

Contributors

Stephen Stich is Professor of Philosophy at Rutgers University.

Michael Tye is Professor of Philosophy at Temple University and at King's College, London.

Andrew Woodfield is Reader in Philosophy at Bristol University.

Aaron Sloman is Professor of Artificial Intelligence and Cognitive Science at the University of Birmingham.

Antony Galton is Lecturer in Computer Science at the University of Exeter.

Stephen Mills is Lecturer in Philosophy at the University of Ulster.

Terence Horgan is Professor of Philosophy at the Memphis State University.

John Tienson is Professor of Philosophy at the Memphis State University.

Niels Ole Bernsen is a member of the Centre of Cognitive Science at Roskilde.

Brian P. McLaughlin is Professor of Philosophy at Rutgers University.

Naturalizing Epistemology: Quine, Simon and the Prospects for Pragmatism

STEPHEN STICH

1. Introduction

In recent years there has been a great deal of discussion about the prospects of developing a 'naturalized epistemology', though different authors tend to interpret this label in quite different ways.[1] One goal of this paper is to sketch three projects that might lay claim to the 'naturalized epistemology' label, and to argue that they are not all equally attractive. Indeed, I'll maintain that the first of the three—the one I'll attribute to Quine—is simply incoherent. There is no way we could get what we want from an epistemological theory by pursuing the project Quine proposes. The second project on my list is a naturalized version of reliabilism. This project is not fatally flawed in the way that Quine's is. However, it's my contention that the sort of theory this project would yield is much less interesting than might at first be thought.

The third project I'll consider is located squarely in the pragmatist tradition. One of the claims I'll make for this project is that if it can be pursued successfully the results will be both more interesting and more useful than the results that might emerge from the reliabilist project. A second claim I'll make for it is that there is some reason to suppose that it *can* be pursued successfully. Indeed, I will argue that for over a decade one version of the project *has* been pursued with considerable success by Herbert Simon and his co-workers in their ongoing attempt to simulate scientific reasoning. In the final section of the paper, I will offer a few thoughts on the various paths Simon's project, and pragmatist naturalized epistemology, might follow in the future.

Before I get on to any of this, however, I had best begin by locating the sort of naturalistic epistemology that I'll be considering in philosophical space. To do this I'll need to say something about how I conceive of epistemology, and to distinguish two

[1] For useful discussions of these various interpretations see Kornblith (1985b) and Kitcher (1992).

1

rather different ideas on what 'naturalizing' might come to. Much of traditional epistemology, and much of contemporary epistemology as well, can be viewed as pursuing one of three distinct though interrelated projects. One of these projects is the assessment of strategies of belief formation and belief revision. Those pursuing this project try to say which ways of building and rebuilding our doxastic house are good ways, which are poor ways, and why. A fair amount of Descartes' epistemological writing falls under this heading, as does much of Bacon's best known work. It is also a central concern in the work of more recent writers like Mill, Carnap and Goodman. A second traditional project aims to provide a definition or characterization of knowledge, explaining how knowledge differs from mere true opinion, as well as from ignorance and error. A third project has as its goal the refutation of the skeptic—the real or imagined opponent who claims that we can't have knowledge or certainty or some other putatively valuable epistemological commodity.[2] Although these three projects are obviously intertwined in various ways, my focus in this paper will be exclusively on the first of the three. The branch of epistemology whose 'naturalization' I'm concerned with here is the branch that attempts to evaluate strategies of belief formation.

Let me turn now to 'naturalizing'. What would it be to 'naturalize' epistemology? There are, I think, two rather different answers that might be given here. I'll call one of them Strong Naturalism and the other Weak Naturalism. What the answers share is the central idea that empirical science has an important role to play in epistemology—that epistemological questions can be investigated and resolved using the methods of the natural or social sciences. The issue over which Strong Naturalism and Weak Naturalism divide is the *extent* to which science can resolve epistemological questions. Strong Naturalism maintains that *all* legitimate epistemological questions are scientific questions, and thus that epistemology can be reduced to or replaced by science. Weak Naturalism, by contrast, claims only that *some* epistemological questions can be resolved by science. According to Weak Naturalism there are some legitimate epistemological questions that are *not* scientific questions and cannot be resolved by scientific research. The sort of epistemological pragmatism that I'll be advocating in this paper is a version of Weak Naturalism. It claims that while some epistemological questions can be resolved by doing science, there is at least one quite fundamental epistemological issue that science cannot settle.

[2] For more on these three projects, see Stich (1990), pp. 1–4.

2. Quine(?)'s Version of Strong Naturalism

The most widely discussed proposal for naturalizing epistemology is the one sketched by Quine in 'Epistemology naturalized' (1969b) and a number of other essays (1969c, 1975). According to Quine,

> [Naturalized epistemology] studies a natural phenomenon, viz. a physical human subject. This human subject is accorded experimentally controlled input—certain patters of irradiation in assorted frequencies, for instance—and in the fullness of time the subject delivers as output a description of the three dimensional external world and its history. The relation between the meagre input and the torrential output is a relation that we are prompted to study for somewhat the same reasons that always prompted epistemology; namely in order to see how evidence relates to theory, and in what ways one's theory of nature transcends any available evidence. (1969b, 82–3)

> The stimulation of his sensory receptors is all the evidence anybody has had to go on, ultimately, in arriving at his picture of the world. Why not just see how this construction really proceeds? Why not settle for psychology? (1969b, 75–6)

There are various ways in which this Quinean proposal might be interpreted. On one reading, Quine is proposing that psychological questions can replace traditional epistemological questions—that instead of asking: How *ought* we to go about forming beliefs and building theories on the basis of evidence? we should ask: How do people actually go about it? And that the answer to this latter, purely psychological question, will tell us what we've really wanted to know all along in epistemology. It will tell us 'how evidence relates to theory'. I'm not at all sure that this is the best interpretation of Quine.[3] What I am sure of is that many people do interpret Quine in this way. I am also sure that on this interpretation, Quine's project is a non-starter.

To see why, let us begin by asking *which* 'physical human subject' or subjects Quine is proposing that we study? Quine doesn't say. Perhaps this is because he supposes that it doesn't much matter, since we're all very much alike. But that is simply not the case.

---

[3] Indeed, in earlier drafts of this paper I attributed the view someone called 'Quine(?)' as a way of emphasizing my uncertainty about the interpretation. But that device survives only in the title of this section; it gets old very quickly.

Consider, for example, those 'physical human subjects' who suffer from Capgras syndrome. These people typically believe that some person close to them has been kidnapped and replaced by a duplicate who looks and behaves almost exactly the same as the original. Some people afflicted with Capgras come to believe that the replacement is not human at all; rather it is a robot with electrical and mechanical components inside. There have even been a few cases reported in which the Capgras sufferer attempted to prove that the 'duplicate' was a robot by attacking it with an axe or a knife in order to expose the wires and transistors concealed beneath the 'skin'. Unfortunately, not even the sight of the quite real wounds and severed limbs that result from these attacks suffice to persuade Capgras patients that the 'duplicate' is real.[4] Now for a Capgras patient, as much as for the rest of us, 'the stimulation of his sensory receptors is all the evidence [he] has had to go on, ultimately, in arriving at his picture of the world'. And psychology might well explore 'how this construction really proceeds'. But surely this process is *not* one that 'we are prompted to study for the same reasons that always prompted epistemology.' For what epistemologists want to know is not how 'evidence relates to theory' in any arbitrary human subject. Rather they want to know how evidence relates to theory in subjects who do a good job of relating them. Among the many actual and possible ways in which evidence might relate to theories, which are the *good* ways and which are the bad ones? That is the question that 'has always prompted epistemology'. And the sort of study that Quine seems to be proposing cannot possibly answer it.

People suffering from Capgras syndrome are, of course, pathological cases. But much the same point can be made about perfectly normal subjects. During the last two decades cognitive psychologists have lavished considerable attention on the study of how normal subjects go about the business of inference and belief revision. Some of the best known findings in this area indicate that in lots of cases people relate evidence to theory in ways that seem normatively dubious to put it mildly (Nisbett and Ross, 1980; Kahneman, Slovic, and Tversky, 1982). More recent work has show that there are significant interpersonal differences in reasoning strategies, some of which can be related to prior education and training (Fong, Krantz and Nisbett, 1986; Nisbett, Fong, Lehman and Cheng, 1987). The Quinean naturalized epistemologist can explore in detail the various ways in which different peo-

---

[4] Foerstl (1990). I am grateful to Lynn Stephens for guiding me to the literature on Capgras syndrome.

ple construct their 'picture of the world' on the basis of the evidence available to them. But he has no way of ranking these quite different strategies for building world descriptions; he has no way of determining which are better and which are worse. And since the Quinean naturalized epistemologist can provide no normative advice whatever, it is more than a little implausible to claim that his questions and projects can replace those of traditional epistemology. We can't 'settle for psychology' because psychology tells us how people *do* reason; it does not (indeed cannot) tell us how they *should*.[5]

3. Reliabilism: Evaluating Reasoning by Studying Reasoners who are Good at Forming True Beliefs

The problem with Quine's proposal is that it doesn't tell us *whose* psychology to 'settle for'. But once this has been noted, there is an obvious proposal for avoiding the problem. If someone wants to improve her chess game, she would be well advised to use the chess strategies that good chess players use. Similarly, if someone wants to improve her reasoning, she would be well advised to use the reasoning strategies that good reasoners use. So rather than studying just anyone, the naturalized epistemologist can focus on those people who do a good job of reasoning. If we can characterize the reasoning strategies that good reasoners employ, then we will have a descriptive theory that has some normative clout.[6]

This, of course, leads directly to another problem. How do we select the people whose reasoning strategies we are going to study? How do we tell the good reasoners from the bad ones? Here there is at least one answer that clearly will *not* do. We can't select people to study by first determining the reasoning strategies that various people use, and then confining our attention to those who use good ones. For that would require that we already know which strategies are good ones; we would be trying to pull ourselves up by our own bootstraps. However, as the analogy with chess suggests, there is a very different way to proceed. We identify good chess players by looking at the consequences of their strategies—

---

[5] For a similar critique of Quine, see Kim (1988).

[6] A number of people have suggested to me that this strategy of studying the reasoning of people who are good at it is what Quine actually had in mind. I find relatively little in Quine's writing to support this interpretation. But I do not pretend to be a serious scholar on such matters. If those who know Quine's work better than I decide that this is what he really intended, I'll be delighted. I can use all the support I can get.

the good players are the ones who win, and the good strategies are the ones that good players use. So we might try to identify good reasoners by looking at the outcome of the reasoning. But this proposal raises further questions: Which 'outcomes' should we look at, and how should we assess them? What counts as 'winning' in epistemology?

One seemingly natural way to proceed here is to focus on *truth*. Reasoning, as Quine stresses, produces 'descriptions of the . . . world and its history'. A bit less behaviouristically, we might say that reasoning produces *theories* that the reasoner comes to *believe*. Some of those theories are true, others are not. And, as the example of the Capgras sufferer's belief makes abundantly clear, false theories can lead to disastrous consequences. So perhaps what we should do is locate reasoners who do a good job at forming *true* beliefs, and try to discover what strategies of reasoning they employ. This project has an obvious affinity with the reliabilist tradition in epistemology. According to reliabilists, truth is a quite basic cognitive virtue, and beliefs are justified if they are produced by a belief forming strategy that generally yields true beliefs. So it would be entirely in order for a naturalistically inclined reliabilist to propose that reasoning strategies should be evaluated by their success in producing true beliefs.[7]

It might be thought that this proposal suffers from something like the same sort of circularity that scuttled the proposal scouted two paragraphs back since we can't identify reasoners who do a good job at producing true theories unless we already know how to distinguish true theories from false ones. On my view, this charge of circularity can't be sustained. There is no overt circularity in the strategy that's been sketched, and the only 'covert' circularity lurking is completely benign, and is to be found in all other accounts of how to tell good reasoning strategies from bad ones. However, I won't pause to set out the arguments rebutting the charge of circularity, since Goldman has already done a fine job of it.[8]

But while this reliabilist project is not viciously circular, it is, I think, much less appealing than might at first be thought. In support of this claim, I'll offer two considerations, one of which I've defended at length elsewhere. The project at hand proposes to dis-

---

[7] The sort of naturalized reliabilism that I am sketching bears an obvious similarity to the psychologically sophisticated reliabilism championed by Alvin Goldman. See, for example, Goldman (1986).

[8] See Goldman (1986) pp. 116–21. In Stich (1990), Section 6.3 I have added a few of my own bells and whistles to Goldman's arguments.

tinguish good reasoning strategies from bad ones on the basis of how well they do at producing true beliefs. But, one might well ask, what's so good about having true beliefs? Why should having true beliefs be taken to be a fundamental goal of cognition? One's answer here must, of course, depend on what one takes true beliefs to be. If, along with Richard Rorty, one thinks that true beliefs are just those that one's community will not challenge when one expresses them, then it is not at all clear why one should want to have true beliefs, unless one values saying what one thinks while avoiding confrontation.[9]

I am not an advocate of Rorty's account of truth, however. On the account I favour, beliefs are mental states of a certain sort that are mapped to propositions (or content sentences) by an intuitively sanctioned 'interpretation function'. Roughly speaking, the proposition to which a belief-like mental state is mapped may be thought of as it's truth condition. The true beliefs are those that are mapped by this function to true propositions, the false beliefs are those that are mapped to false propositions. However, it is my contention that the intuitively sanctioned function that determines truth conditions—the one that maps beliefs to propositions—is both arbitrary and idiosyncratic. There are lots of other functions mapping the same class of mental states to propositions in quite different ways. And these alternative functions assign different (albeit counter-intuitive) truth conditions. The class of beliefs mapped to true propositions by these counter-intuitive functions may be slightly different, or very different from the class of beliefs mapped to true propositions by the intuitive function. So, using the counter-intuitive functions we can define classes of beliefs that might be labelled TRUE* beliefs, TRUE** beliefs, and so on. A TRUE* belief is just one that is mapped to a true proposition by a counter-intuitive mapping function. Yet many of the alternative functions are no more arbitrary or idiosyncratic than the intuitively sanctioned function. Indeed, the only special feature that the intuitively sanctioned function has is that it is the one we happened to have been bequeathed by our language and culture. If all of this is right, then it is hard to see why we should prefer a system of reasoning that typically yields true beliefs over a system that typically yields TRUE* beliefs. The details on all of this, and the supporting arguments, have been set out elsewhere (Stich, 1990, Ch. 5; 1991a; 1991b). Since there is not space enough to recon-

---

[9] This is, of course, no more than a caricature of Rorty's view. The full view defies easy summary. See Rorty (1979), Ch. 8; (1982), pp. xiii–xlvii; (1988).

struct them here, let me offer a rather different sort of argument to challenge the idea that good reasoning strategies are those that typically yield true beliefs.

If one wants to play excellent chess, one would be well advised to use the strategies used by the best players in their best games. Of course, it *may* be possible to do even better than the best players of the past. One can always hope. But surely a good first step would be to figure out the strategies that the best players were using at the height of their power. For barring cosmic accident, those are likely to be very good strategies indeed. Now suppose we were to try to apply this approach not to chess strategies but to reasoning strategies. Whose reasoning would we study?

Here opinions might differ, of course. But I suspect that most of us would have the great figures of the history of science high on our list. Aristotle, Newton, Dalton, Mendel—these are some of the names that would be on my list of Grand Masters at the 'game' of reasoning. If one is a reliabilist, however, there is something quite odd about this list. For in each case the theories for which the thinker is best known, the theories they produced at the height of their cognitive powers, have turned out not to be true. Nor is this an idiosyncratic feature of this particular collection of thinkers. It is a commonplace observation in the history of science that much of the best work of many of the best scientific thinkers of the past has turned out to be mistaken. In some cases historical figures seem to be getting 'closer' to the truth than their predecessors. But in other cases they seem to be getting further away. And in many cases this notoriously obscure notion of 'closer to the truth' seems to make little sense.

The conclusion that I would draw here is that if we adopt the strategy of locating good reasoners by assessing the *truth* of their best products, we will end up studying the wrong class of thinkers. For some of the best examples of human reasoning that we know of do not typically end up producing true theories. If we want to know how to do a good job of reasoning—if we want to be able to do it the way Newton did it—then we had better not focus our attention exclusively on thinkers who got the right answer.

4. Pragmatism: There are no Special Cognitive Goals or Virtues

The project sketched in the previous section might be thought of as having two parts. The first part was entirely normative. It was claimed that truth was a quite special cognitive virtue, and that achieving true beliefs was the goal in terms of which strategies of reasoning should be evaluated. The second part was empirical. Having decided that good cognition was cognition that produced true belief, we try to identify people who excel by that measure, and then study the way they go about the business of reasoning. Using the terminology suggested in Section 1, the project is a version of Weak Naturalism. Science, broadly construed, can tell us which reasoners do a good job at producing true beliefs, and what strategies of reasoning they exploit. But science can't either confirm or disconfirm the initial normative step. Science can't tell us by what standard strategies of reasoning *should* be evaluated. The critique of the project that I offered in the previous section was aimed entirely at the normative component. It is, I argued, far from obvious that producing true beliefs is the standard against which strategies of reasoning should be measured.

But if truth is not to be the standard in epistemology, what is? The answer that I favour is one that plays a central role in the pragmatist tradition. For pragmatists, there are *no* special cognitive or epistemological values. There are just *values*. Reasoning, inquiry and cognition are viewed as tools that we use in an effort to achieve what we value. And like any other tools, they are to be assessed by determining how good a job they do at achieving what we value. So on the pragmatist view, the good cognitive strategies for a person to use are those that are likely to lead to the states of affairs that he or she finds intrinsically valuable. This is, of course, a thoroughly relativistic account of good reasoning. For if two people have significantly different intrinsic values, then it may well turn out that a strategy of reasoning that is good for one may be quite poor for the other. There is, in the pragmatist tradition, a certain tendency to down play or even deny the epistemic relativism to which pragmatism leads. But on my view this failure of nerve is a great mistake. Relativism in the evaluation of reasoning strategies is no more worrisome than relativism in the evaluation of diets or investment strategies or exercise programmes. The fact that different strategies of reasoning may be good for different people is a fact of life that pragmatists should accept with equanimity.[10]

As I envision it, the pragmatist project for assessing reasoning strategies proceeds as follows. First, we must determine which goal or goals are of interest for the assessment at hand. We must decide what it is that we want our reasoning to achieve. This step, of course, is fundamentally normative. Empirical inquiry may be of help in making the decision, but science alone will not tell you

---

[10] For more on pragmatism and relativism, see Stich (1990), Section 6.2.

what your goals are. Thus the pragmatist's project, like the reliabilist's, is a version of Weak Naturalism. The second step is to locate people who have done a good job at achieving the goal or goals selected. The third step—and typically it is here that most of the hard work comes in—is to discover the strategies of reasoning and inquiry that these successful subjects have used in achieving the specified goal. Just as in the case of chess, the expectation is that if we can discover the strategies used by those who have done a good job at achieving the goals we value, these will be good strategies for us to use as well. But we need not assume that they are the best possible strategies. It may well be that once we gain some understanding of the strategies used by people who have excelled in achieving the specified goals, we may find ways of improving on their strategies. Exploring the possibility of improving on the actual strategies of successful cognitive agents is the fourth step in the pragmatist project.

5. Herbert Simon's Computational Pragmatism

The pragmatist project sketched in the previous section is of a piece with the epistemological theory I defended in *The Fragmentation of Reason*. Shortly after that book was completed I was delighted to discover that for more than two decades Herbert Simon and his colleagues had been hard at work on a project that had all the essential features of the one I have proposed. They had long been practising what I had only recently started to preach.[11]

Simon's project is an ambitious research programme in artificial intelligence. He characterizes the project, rather provocatively, as an attempt to construct a 'logic of scientific discovery'. The 'logic' that Simon seeks would be an explicit set of principles for reasoning and the conduct of inquiry which, when followed systematically, will result in the production of good scientific hypotheses and theories. As is generally the case in artificial intelligence, the princi-

[11] The literature in this area is extensive and growing quickly. While Simon is clearly a seminal figure, many others have done important work. In much of what follows, 'Simon' should be read as shorthand for 'Simon and his co-workers'. Perhaps the best place to get an overview of Simon's work in this area is in Langley, Simon, Bradshaw and Zytkow (1987). For a review of more recent work see Shrager and Langley (1990b) and the other essays in Shrager and Langley (1990a). Other useful sources include Simon (1966), Simon (1973), Buchanan (1983), Kulkarni and Simon (1988), Zytkow and Simon (1988), Thagard (1988) and Kulkarni and Simon (1990).

ples must be explicit enough to be programmed on a computer. Simon and his co-workers don't propose to construct their logic of discovery by relying on *a priori* principles or philosophical arguments about how science should proceed; their approach is much more empirical. To figure out how to produce good scientific theories, they study and try to simulate what good scientists do. In some ways their project is quite similar to 'expert systems' studies in AI. The initial goal is to produce a computational simulation of the reasoning of people who are 'experts' at doing science.

Though Simon does not stress the point, he acknowledges that a largely parallel project might be undertaken with the goal of simulating the reasoning of some other class of 'experts'. We might, for example, focus on the reasoning of people who have done outstanding work in history, or in literary criticism, or in theology. In some of these cases (or all of them) we might end up with pretty much the same principles of reasoning. But then again, we might not. It might well turn out that different strategies of reasoning work best in different domains. The choice of which group of reasoners to study—and ultimately, the choice of which strategy to use in one's own reasoning—is the initial normative step in Simon's pragmatic project.

Having decided that the reasoning he wants to study is the sort that leads to success in science, the second step in Simon's project is to identify people who have achieved scientific success. As a practical matter, of course, this is easy enough. There is a fair amount of agreement on who the great scientists of the past have been. But when pressed to provide some justification for the scientists he selects, Simon (only half jokingly) suggests the following way to 'operationalize' the choice: Go to the library and get a collection of the most widely used basic textbooks in various fields. Then sit down and make a list of the people whose pictures appear in the textbooks. Those are the people whose reasoning we should study. Though I rather doubt that Simon has ever actually done this, the joke makes a serious point. The criterion of success that Simon is using is not the *truth* of the theories that various scientists produce. To be a successful scientist, as Simon construes the notion, is to be famous enough to get one's picture in the textbooks.

With a list of successful scientists at hand, the really challenging part of Simon's project can begin. The goal is to build a computational simulation of the cognitive processes that led successful scientists to their most celebrated discoveries. To do this, a fair amount of historical information is required, since optimally the input to the simulation should include as much as can be discovered about the data available to the scientist who is the target of the simulation, along with information about the received theories and background assumptions that the scientist was likely to bring to the project. As with other efforts at cognitive simulation, there is a variety of evidence that can be used to confirm or disconfirm the simulation as it develops. First, of course, the simulation must end up producing the same law or theory that the target scientist produced. Second, the simulation should go through intermediate steps parallel to those that the scientist went through in the course of making his or her discovery. In some cases, laboratory note-books and other historical evidence provide a quite rich portrait of the inferential steps (and mis-steps) that the target scientist made along the way. But in most cases the details of the scientist's reasoning are at best very sketchy. In an effort to generate more data against which the simulation can be tested, Simon and his co-workers have used laboratory studies of problem solving and 're-discovery' in which talented students are asked to come up with a law or theory that will capture a set of data, where the data provided are at least roughly similar to the data available to the target scientist. While they are working, the students are asked to 'think out loud' and explain the various steps they make. The problems are often very hard ones, and relatively few students succeed. But the protocols generated by the successful students can be used as another source of data against which simulation programs can be tested (Kulkarni and Simon, 1988; Dunbar, 1989: Qin and Simon, 1990).

It should be stressed that there is no *a priori* guarantee that Simon's research programme will be successful. There is a long tradition which insists that scientific creativity, indeed all creativity, is a deeply mysterious process, far beyond the reach of computational theories. And even if we don't accept the mystery theory of creativity, it is entirely possible that efforts to simulate the reasoning which led one or another important scientist to a great discovery will fail. The only way to silence these concerns is to deliver the goods. It is also possible that while each individual scientist's reasoning can be simulated successfully, each case is different. There might be no interesting regularities that all cases of successful scientific reasoning share. Perhaps successful scientific reasoning is discipline specific, and different strategies of reasoning are successful in different disciplines. Worse still, it might turn out that no two successful scientists exploit the same strategies. Styles of successful reasoning might be entirely idiosyncratic. Having noted these concerns, however, I should also note that it doesn't look like things *are* turning out this way. While there is still lots of work to be done, Simon and his group have produced impressive simulations of Kepler's discovery of the his third law, Kreb's discovery of the urea cycle, and a variety of other important scientific discoveries. While some of the heuristics used in these simulations are specific to a particular scientific domain, none are specific to a particular problem, and many appear to be domain independent (Kulkarni and Simon, 1990, Section 5). So, though the jury is still out, I think it is entirely reasonable to view Simon's successes to date as an excellent beginning on the sort of pragmatist naturalization of epistemology that I advocated in the previous section. In the final section of this paper, I want to consider some of the ways in which Simon-style pragmatist projects may develop in the future.

6. Beyond History's Best: Future Projects for Naturalistic Pragmatism

The project of simulating successful scientific reasoning is the one that has preoccupied Simon and his co-workers up until now. However, once some substantial success has been achieved along these lines—and it is my reading of the situation that we are now at just about that stage—it becomes possible to explore some new, and very exciting territory. As the historical record indicates, important discoveries are often slow in coming and they frequently involve steps that later come to be seen as unnecessary or unfruitful. To the extent that simulations like Simon's have as their goal understanding the details of the psychological process that lead to discoveries, it is, of course, a virtue if they explore blind alleys just where the scientists they were modelling did. However, if we want a normative rather than a descriptive theory of discovery, it is no particular virtue to mimic the mistaken steps and wasted efforts of gifted scientists. Thus rather than aiming to describe the cognitive strategies of gifted scientists, we might aspire to *improve* on those strategies. By tinkering with the programme—or, more interestingly, by developing a substantive theory of how and why they work—we may well be able to design programmes that do *better* than real people, including very gifted and highly trained people, be they important historical figures or clever students in laboratory studies of reasoning. I think that to a certain extent this sort of tinkering and theory driven improvement is already a part of Simon's project, though it is often not clearly separated from the process of modeling actual discovery. The process of improvement can be pursued along several rather different lines. What distinguishes them is the sort of *constraints* that the computational model takes to be important. In the remaining pages of this paper I want to sketch some of the constraints that might be imposed or ignored, and consider the sorts of projects that might ensue.

A first division turns on how much importance we attach to the idea that normative rules and strategies of reasoning have to be usable by human beings. To the extent that we take that constraint seriously, we will not propose strategies of reasoning that are difficult or impossible for a human cognitive system. Our normative theory will respect the limitations imposed by human psychology and human hardware. A natural label for this project might be *Human Epistemology*. Of course, the more our normative theory of Human Epistemology respects the limits and idiosyncrasies of human cognition, the closer it will resemble the descriptive theory of good reasoning. But there is no reason to think that the two will collapse. For it may well be the case that there are readily learnable and readily usable strategies of reasoning that would improve on those that were in fact used in the 'exemplary' cases of scientific discovery. In order pursue Human Epistemology in a serious way we will need detailed information about the nature and the rigidity of constraints on human cognition. And the only way to get this information is to do the relevant empirical work. This is yet another way in which the sort of naturalized epistemology that I am advocating requires input from empirical science.[12]

What happens if we are not much concerned with constraining our epistemological system by taking account of the facts of human cognition? We aren't free of all constraints, since the commitment to construct theories of scientific discovery that are explicit enough to be *programmable* imposes its own constraints. The theories we build must be implementable with available hardware and available software. But, of course, there are lots of things that available systems can do quite easily that human brains cannot do at all. So if we are prepared to ignore the facts about human cognition, we are likely to get a very different family of normative theories of scientific discovery. In recent work, Clark Glymour has introduced the term *Android Epistemology*, and I think that would be an ideal label to borrow for normative theories like these.

If there were more space available, I would spend it exploring the prospects for Android Epistemology. For it seems to me that they are very exciting prospects indeed. What is slowly emerging from the work of Simon's group, and from the work of other

[12] For some interesting studies aimed at discovering how much plasticity there is in human reasoning, see the papers in Nisbett (1993), Part VI.

groups focusing on related problems, is, in effect, a *technology of discovery*. We are beginning to see to the development of artefacts that can discover useful laws, useful concepts and useful theories. It is, of course, impossible to know how successful these efforts will ultimately be. But I, for one, would not be at all surprised if future historians viewed this work as a major juncture in human intellectual history.

Let me return to the domain of Human Epistemology. For there is one more distinction that needs to be drawn here. Once again the notion of constraints provides a convenient way to draw the distinction. One of the facts about real human cognizers is that they are embedded in a social context. They get information and support from other people, they compete with others in various ways, and their work is judged by others. Many of the rewards for their efforts come from the surrounding society as the result of these judgements. In building our *Normative Human Epistemology* we may choose to take account of these factors or to ignore them.

In their work to date, Simon and his colleagues have largely chosen to ignore these social constraints. And for good reason. Things are complicated enough already, without trying to see how well our simulations do when competing with other simulations in a complex social environment. None the less, I think there may ultimately be a great deal to learn by taking the social constraints seriously, and exploring what we might label *Social Epistemology*. For example, Philip Kitcher (1990) has recently tried to show that the likely payoff of pursuing long shots in science—the expected utility of working hard to defend implausible theories—depends in important ways on the distribution of intellectual labour in the rest of the community. I think there is reason to hope that if we take seriously the idea of building epistemological theories for socially embedded cognitive agents we may begin to find ways in which the organization of the inquiring community itself may be improved. We may find better ways to fund research, channel intellectual effort, deal with dishonesty and distribute rewards. As a pragmatist, I can think of no finer future for epistemology.[13]

[13] Earlier versions of this paper were presented at the Conference on Methods at the New School for Social Research, the Southern Society for Philosophy and Psychology, the Australasian Association for Philosophy and the conference on Philosophy and Cognitive Science at the University of Birmingham. I am grateful to the audiences at all these meetings for many helpful suggestions. Thanks are also due to Peter Klein for extended comments on the penultimate version of the paper, and to Paul Lodge for help in preparing the final version of the manuscript.

15

References

Buchanan, B. 1983. 'Mechanizing the search for explanatory hypotheses', in P. Asquith and T. Nichols (eds), *PSA 1982*, Vol. 2. East Lansing, MI: Philosophy of Science Association.

Dunbar, K. 1989. 'Scientific reasoning strategies in a simulated molecular genetics environment', *Proceedings of the Eleventh Annual Meeting of the Cognitive Science Society* Ann Arbor, MI: Erlbaum.

Foerstl, H. 1990. 'Capgras' delusion', *Comprehensive Psychiatry*, **31**, 447–449.

Fong, G., Krantz, D. and Nisbett, R. 1986. 'The effects of statistical training on thinking about everyday problems', *Cognitive Psychology* **18**, 253–292.

Goldman, A. 1986. *Epistemology and Cognition*. Cambridge, MA: Harvard University Press.

Kahneman, D., Slovic, P. and Tversky, A. (eds) 1982. *Judgment Under Uncertainty*. Cambridge: Cambridge University Press.

Kim, J. 1988. 'What is "Naturalized Epistemology?"' *Philosophical Perspectives*, **2**, 381–405.

Kitcher, P. 1990. 'The division of cognitive labor', *Journal of Philosophy*, **87**, 5–22.

Kitcher, P. 1992. 'The naturalists return', *Philosophical Review*, **101**, 53–114.

Kornblith, H. (ed.) 1985a. *Naturalizing Epistemology*, Cambridge, MA: MIT Press.

Kornblith, H. 1985b. 'What is naturalistic epistemology?' in Kornblith (1985a), 1–13.

Kulkarni, D. and Simon, H. 1988. 'The processes of scientific discovery: The strategy of experimentation', *Cognitive Science*, **12**, 139–175.

Kulkarni, D. and Simon, H. 1990. 'Experimentation in Machine Discovery', in Shrager and Langley (1990a).

Langley, P., Simon, H., Bradshaw, G. and Zytkow, J. 1987. *Scientific Discovery: Computational Explorations of the Creative Processes*.

Nisbett, R. (ed.) 1993. *Rules for Reasoning*. Hillsdale, NJ: Erlbaum.

Nisbett, R. and Ross, L. 1980. *Human Inference*. Englewood Cliffs, NJ: Prentice-Hall.

Nisbett, R., Fong, G., Lehman, D. and Cheng, P. 1987. 'Teaching reasoning', *Science*, **238**, 625–631.

Qin, Y, and Simon, H. 1990. 'Laboratory replication of scientific discovery processes', *Cognitive Science*, **14**, 281–312.

Quine, W. 1969a. *Ontological Relativity and Other Essays*. New York: Columbia University Press.

Quine, W. 1969b. 'Epistemology naturalized', in Quine (1969a), 69–90. Reprinted in Kornblith (1985a).

Quine, W. 1969c. 'Natural kinds', in Quine (1969a), 114–138. Reprinted in Kornblith (1985a).

Quine, W. 1975. 'The nature of natural knowledge', in S. Guttenplan (ed.) *Mind and language*. Oxford: Clarendon Press.

Rorty, R. 1979. *Philosophy and the Mirror of Nature*. Princeton: Princeton University Press.

Rorty, R. 1982. *Consequences of Pragmatism*. Minneapolis: University of Minnesota Press.

Rorty, R. 1988. 'Representation, social practice, and truth', *Philosophical Studies*, **54**, 215–228.

Shrager, J. and Langley, P. (eds) 1990a. *Computational Models of Scientific Discovery and Theory Formation*. San Mateo, CA: Morgan Kaufmann Publishers.

Shrager, J. and Langley, P. 1990b. 'Computational approaches to scientific discovery', in Shrager and Langley (1990a).

Simon, H. 1966. 'Scientific discovery and the psychology of problem solving', in R. Colodny (ed.), *Mind and Cosmos: Essays in Contemporary Science and Philosophy*, Pittsburgh: University of Pittsburgh Press.

Simon, H. 1973. 'Does scientific discovery have a logic?' *Philosophy of Science*, **40**, 471–480.

Stich, S. 1990. *The Fragmentation of Reason*. Cambridge, MA: MIT Press.

Stich, S. 1991a. *"The Fragmentation of Reason* – Precis of two chapters', *Philosophy and Phenomenological Research*, **51**, 179–183.

Stich, S. 1991b. 'Evaluating cognitive strategies: A reply to Cohen, Goldman, Harman and Lycan', *Philosophy and Phenomenological Research*, **51**, 207-213.

Thagard, P. 1988. *Computational Philosophy of Science*. Cambridge, MA: MIT Press.

Zytkow, J. and Simon, H. 1988. 'Normative systems of discovery and logic of search', *Synthese*, **74**, 65–90.

Blindsight, the Absent Qualia Hypothesis, and the Mystery of Consciousness

MICHAEL TYE

One standard objection to the view that phenomenal experience is functionally determined is based upon what has come to be called 'The Absent Qualia Hypothesis', the idea that there could be a person or a machine that was functionally exactly like us but that felt or consciously experienced nothing at all (see Block, 1980; Block and Fodor, 1980; Campbell, 1980; Nagel, 1980). Advocates of this hypothesis typically maintain that we can easily imagine possible systems that meet the appropriate functional specifications but that intuitively lack any phenomenal consciousness. Ned Block (1980), for example, asks us to suppose that a billion Chinese people are each given a two-way radio with which to communicate with one another and with an artificial (brainless) body. The movements of the body are controlled by the radio signals, and the signals themselves are made in accordance with instructions the Chinese people receive from a vast display in the sky which is visible to all of them. The instructions are such that the participating Chinese people together realize whatever programs the functionalist supposes underlie human phenomenal experience.

The usual functionalist reply to imaginary examples of this sort is to suggest that it is not at all obvious that the given system really would lack feelings and experiences (Lycan 1987). After all, in the case of the China-body system, if we were to translate the system's outputs and engage it in conversation, we would get precisely the responses we would expect from a system that was genuinely feeling pain and other experiential states. Our initial intuition that the system does not feel anything may be traced to our relative size. Just as a tiny, intelligent being living inside Block's head might well be unable to see the forest for the trees and leap to the false conclusion that Block didn't feel anything, so too we have a highly restricted perspective that easily deceives us into thinking that the China-body system could not undergo phenomenal experiences.

Who is right? It seems to me radically unclear. In my view, intuitions about what we can or cannot imagine in cases like the one above are unstable and not to be trusted (see Tye, 1986).

Arguing for (or against) the Absent Qualia Hypothesis on the basis of imaginability is a misguided strategy.

Recently, a number of philosophers have turned their attention to some examples from real life that seem to conform, at least in part, to the requirements of the Absent Qualia Hypothesis (see, for example, Heil, 1983; Dennett, 1991; McGinn, 1991). These examples concern a condition known as blindsight that has been extensively studied in the last decade in psychology. People with blindsight have large blind areas or scotoma in their visual fields, due to brain damage in the post-genniculate region (typically the occipital cortex), and yet, under certain circumstances, they can issue accurate statements and draw accurate pictures with respect to the contents of those areas. In short, given appropriate instructions, they can apparently function in much the same way as normally sighted subjects, with regard to the blind areas in their visual fields, without there being anything experiential or phenomenally conscious going on. Blindsight subjects, then, are apparently unconscious automata with regard to some stimuli while remaining fully conscious with regard to others.

How is blindsight best understood? Do we genuinely have here some real life cases that are, in any way, relevant to the Absent Qualia Hypothesis (or a restricted version of that hypothesis)— cases of people, some of whose inner states are functionally similar to those of normal subjects while lacking intrinsic phenomenal features? Or is their impairment of a different sort? If so, just what is it that blindsight subjects are lacking? And what can reflection on blindsight tell us, if anything, about the alleged mystery of consciousness? These are the questions I shall be addressing.

My paper is divided into four sections. I begin by discussing three sorts of visual agnosia which may usefully be compared with blindsight, and I lay out a psychological model proposed by Martha Farah (1991) for understanding these visual impairments. In Section II, I briefly review some of the main experimental findings in connection with blindsight, and I present an empirical hypothesis, which makes use of Farah's model, for explaining them. In Section III, I draw out the consequences of my discussion of blindsight and visual agnosia for the Absent Qualia Hypothesis. In the final section, I make some remarks on the mystery of consciousness.

I

Higher level vision begins with the combining of local elements of the visual field into contours, regions, and/or surfaces. The first thing that can go wrong, then, in higher level vision is this process of grouping. The resulting impairment is known as apperceptive agnosia (in the narrow sense). It is typically brought about by damage to the occipital lobes and surrounding regions (by, e.g., carbon monoxide poisoning). These patients often have roughly normal visual fields, so their perception of colour, brightness, and local contour is adequate. But they are strikingly impaired in the ability to recognize, match, or even copy simple shapes as well as more complicated figures.[1] In general, they have great difficulty in performing any visual tasks that require combining information across local regions of the visual field.[2] For example, when shown *Figure 1*, one patient consistently read it as 7415.[3]

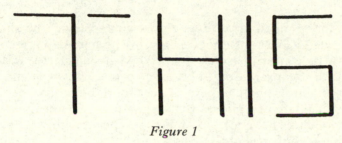

Figure 1

Evidently he was unable to see two parts of a line with a small gap as parts of a single line.[4]

One reasonable hypothesis, then, is that there is a stage in vision in which representations of the local elements of the visual field are combined or grouped into an overall representation of the surfaces visible from the given point of view. This latter representation, which specifies lines, edges, ridges, and other surface features, is a vital foundation for nearly all higher level visual processing. It seems

[1] Movement of shapes sometimes helps these patients to identify them. See, for example, R. Efron (1968, p. 159).

[2] They do better at identifying real objects (e.g., toothbrushes, safety pins), than simple shapes. However, their improved performance here is based on *inferences* from clues provided by color, texture, reflectance.

[3] The patient made this identification by tracing around the figure with movements of his hand and relying on local continuity. See here Landis *et al.* (1982).

[4] Patients with this impairment are often classified with those who have a disorder called 'simultanagnosia'. In reality, the syndromes are distinct, however. Moreover, to confuse matters further, the term 'simultanagnosia' has been used to cover two different syndromes, as we shall shortly see. The classification I shall be using is the one suggested by Farah (1991).

plausible to suppose that it has the structure of a grouped array like Marr's 2 1/2-D sketch (Marr, 1982), the cells of which are devoted to specific lines of sight relative to the viewer (with different cells devoted to different lines).[5] As such, it does contain information about local features of the visual field too, e.g., colour, texture, and orientation.

There is no clear evidence that the process of grouping is cognitively penetrable. So, for example, the patient above, even though he was much more familiar with the word 'THIS' than the number sequence 7415, had no tendency to see the pattern as a word. In general, impairments in grouping seem to derive wholly from physical properties of the stimuli, e.g., whether there is a break in a line, whether the presented lines are rounded or straight, and so on.

Now the grouped array does not itself represent the shapes of any objects visible to the viewer (e.g., whether they are cubes or spheres). Its concern is solely with the visible surfaces. Indeed, at this level in the processing there is no segmentation of the visible scene into objects at all. What are needed in the next levels of processing, then, are procedures that generate viewpoint independent representations of the visible objects' shapes together with procedures that identify the objects' locations.

Ungerleider and Mishkin (1982) have hypothesized that the former procedures occur in the ventral system, which runs from area

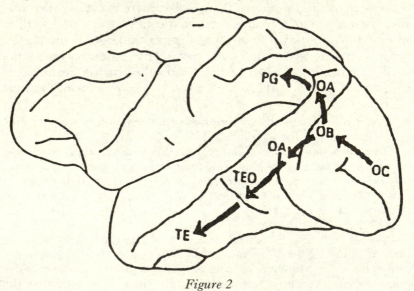

Figure 2

[5] For more on arrays, see my *The Imagery Debate* (1991b).

OC (primary visual cortex) through area TEO to the inferior temporal lobe. This system is concerned with the identification of what is present. The latter procedures are handled by a second system in the brain known as the dorsal system. It runs from circumstriate area OB to OA and then on to PG (in the parietal lobe). The two systems together enable us to recognize objects when they appear in different positions in the visual field.

Dorsal simultanagnosia is an impairment in the dorsal system. Patients with this impairment frequently have full visual fields, but they seem blind with respects to parts of the field. They can recognize familiar objects, but they typically can only see one at a time. For example, one patient was shown the picture in *Figure 3* for 2 seconds. She reported that she saw mountains. When shown

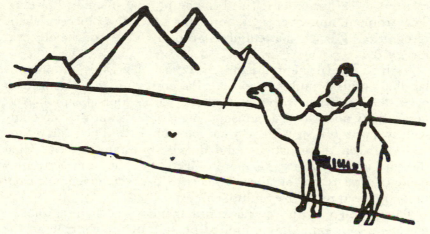

Figure 3

the same picture again for 2 seconds, she said that she saw a man. She apparently did not see the mountains or the camel, and she gave no indication that she realized it was the same picture. When presented with the picture for 30 seconds, she described it accurately, but she reported that she never saw it 'whole'. Instead she saw 'bits' of it that 'faded out' (Tyler, 1968). Another patient, who was watching the end of a cigarette held between his lips, is reported (by Hecaen and Ajuriaguerra, 1974) to have been unable to see the flame from a match offered to him one or two inches from the cigarette.

The impairment here is clearly one of attention. Dorsal simultanagnosics have a severe attentional defect, one that results in 'tunnel' vision and precludes them from seeing unattended objects at all. The strongest evidence for the latter claim is this: when

23

experimenters made sudden threatening movements towards the subjects while their attention was focussed elsewhere in the field of view, they did not react at all (see Godwin-Austen, 1965). However, the normal response was brought about by the same movements within the focus of attention.

Since dorsal simultanagnosics can only attend to one object at a time, they cannot recognize spatial relationships between presented objects even though they can recognize what those objects are, given appropriate shifts of attention. Nor can they adequately localize seen objects. This is shown by their failure to point correctly at the objects or to reach successfully for them.[6]

What these facts suggest is that dorsal simultanagnosia is an impairment in the dorsal system, in which attention is severely limited in its scope and not easily disengaged. The grouped array referred to earlier is itself filled in the normal manner, however. The problem, moreover, is not one that precludes object or shape recognition. For when attention is properly focussed, the object is recognized.

A third impairment arising in higher level vision may be labelled 'ventral simultanagnosia'. Patients with this impairment have defects in their ventral systems. Like dorsal simultanagnosics, they do well at recognising single objects but they do badly with two or more, or with very complex objects.[7] The main difference between these patients and dorsal simultanagnosics is that they are able to *see* two or more objects. So, they can accurately point to, and reach for, these objects. Moreover, given sufficient time, they can recognize multiple objects.

The problem with ventral simultanagnosics, then, is one of object recognition.[8] Only a limited portion of the contents of the grouped array can be recognized in the period of time normally required for object recognition. So, ventral simultanagnosics have no impairments in the attention system or in the processes responsible for the grouped array. Their deficit is one of slowed object recognition.

The fact that ventral and dorsal simultanagnosia are doubly dissociable seems to show that the attentional system and the object recognition system cannot be arranged in series—neither can pro-

[6] The failure to localize stimuli, even when they are seen, has been labelled 'visual disorientation'.

[7] Their reading is also severely impaired.

[8] For ease of exposition, the term 'object' here, and in what follows, is used broadly to include shapes. So, when I refer to the object recognition system, I have in mind the system or systems which enable us to recognize cubes, cylinders, and cones as well as mice, men, and mountains.

vide necessary input to the other. However, some evidence seems to support the opposite view. The impairment in dorsal simultanagnosia is connected with the number of objects. So, it appears that the input to the attention system has already been examined at some level by the object recognition system. Also, ventral simultanagnosics improve their performance, given appropriate spatial cuing. So, paradoxically, it appears that the input to the object recognition system can be operated upon first by attention.

Martha Farah (1991, pp. 150–153) has proposed that these facts may be explained by the architecture shown below in which the grouped array is operated upon directly by a spatial attention system and an object recognition system in parallel. The suggestion basically is that the spatial attention system is set into operation either by top-down instructions (e.g., a decision to pay attention to a certain part of the visual field) or by bottom up factors (e.g., the movement or onset of a stimulus). This system, then, selects portions of the grouped array, the result being that stimuli represented in those portions are more likely to be detected, and are also more likely to be recognized, by the object recognition system. It seems plausible to suppose that the process of selection here involves adding activation to portions of the array. As shown in *Figure 4*, the object recognition system is also hypothesized to interact with the contents of the array so that activation in certain portions of the array may increase during the course of recognition.

We can now explain how ventral simultanagnosics are able to recognize objects at spatially cued locations, among many other objects at different locations, without significant difficulty. In these cases, the spatial attention system adds activation to the relevant parts of the array, thereby causing the object recognition system to process those parts first. Since ventral simultanagnosics have object recognition systems which are capable of recognizing single objects, the object at the spatially cued location will be identified.

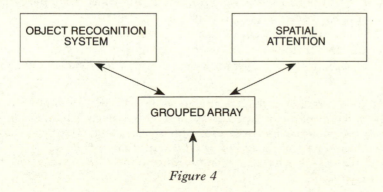

Figure 4

We can also now explain one of the most puzzling facts about dorsal simultanagnosia, namely why it is linked to the number of objects present. The object recognition system, in operating on the array, will cause certain portions of it to become more active—portions corresponding to objects. The activity in these portions will cause the spatial attention system to select them. So, attention will be focussed on regions of the array for which there are corresponding objects. The defect in the spatial attention system is such that attention then stays stuck to one of these regions ('sticky' attention, as Farah calls it). So, only a single region corresponding to an object will be sufficiently activated for the object recognition system to deliver a result. Once attention is disengaged from this region it can then operate on other regions, but the same problem arises again. So, only individual objects are recognized without any awareness of their spatial relationships to one another.[9]

Let us now consider how this model might be applied to understanding blind sight.

II

Blindsight subjects have a definite portion of the field with respect to which they take themselves to be blind. These portions can be marked out by slowly changing the location of a spot of light in the visual field, and by asking the subjects whether they can still experience it. Why are they apparently lacking consciousness with respect to their blind areas? If Farah's model is along the right lines, then one important requirement in the production of visual experience in human beings is that the spatial attention system select the contents of a portion of the grouped array for further processing by the object recognition system. It might be supposed, then, that with blindsight subjects, there is an impairment which prevents their spatial attention systems from *locking on* to a certain portion of the grouped array. So, the contents of that part of the array never get selected by the attentional system.

This proposal, however, cannot be reconciled with what we know about the location of brain damage in blindsight subjects. Let me explain. One major subcortical pathway from the eyes into

---

[9] It should be noted that, in the above framework, attention operates on the contents of the grouped array, and not relatively late in visual processing on object-based representations, as is standardly assumed. Notwithstanding this fact, Farah (1991, p. 153) maintains that it can explain the data that have been adduced in support of object-based theories of attention.

the brain is known as the *geniculo-striate* pathway. It runs from the retina to the lateral-geniculate nucleus of the thalamus, and then from there into the occipital lobe. Patients with blindsight have damage to this pathway. By contrast, patients with defects in their spatial attention systems have damage in the parieto-occipital regions. So, given that the grouped array itself is located in the occipital lobe,[10] the hypothesis that blindsight is due to an impairment in the linkage between the spatial attention system and the grouped array appears to locate the problem in the wrong place, namely beyond the geniculo-striate pathway.[11]

There is a second possible approach to blindsight that is consistent with Farah's model. We saw earlier that in the case of apperceptive agnosics, there is an impairment in the grouping processes which produce the grouped array, an impairment that leaves the array with only partial representation of non-local features in the visual field. Blindsight, I tentatively suggest, is a similar but more extreme impairment, one that leaves a significant portion of the grouped array completely without any representation of either local or non-local features. As a result, blindsight subjects are not conscious at all of the contents of their scotoma, whereas apperceptive agnosics retain consciousness of purely local features.

This proposal is consistent with the location of brain damage in blindsight subjects. What remain to be explained, of course, are the discriminatory capacities these subjects retain with respect to the contents of their scotoma. In particular, psychologists have been puzzled by the fact that accurate guesses can be made with respect to such things as presence, position, orientation, and movement of visual stimuli, and the related fact that, when a pattern is flashed into the blind field, it attracts the eye towards it just as with normally sighted subjects. There is also the intriguing phenomenon known as completion.

Under certain special conditions, if stimuli are presented to both the blind and the intact parts of the visual field, both will be registered. By contrast, if the stimulus is presented just to the blind field, nothing is reported. One psychologist who has exploited this approach to blindsight is Tony Marcel.[12] The method Marcel used

---

[10] This is suggested not only by the location of brain damage in apperceptive agnosics but also by positron emission tomography (PET) scanning. See here Stephen Kosslyn and Oliver Roenig (1992, pp. 67–70).

[11] The same objection can be raised to the hypothesis that blindsight is due to a defect in the functioning of the mechanism of introspective awareness. I should perhaps add here that it is important not to confuse introspective awareness with respect to visual experiences with the opera-

was to induce after-images for shapes with a bright photoflash. He then asked his two subjects (T & G) to draw what they saw. The results are shown in *Figure 5*:

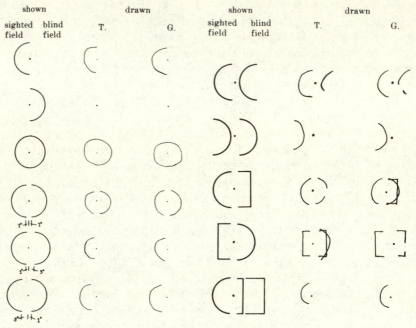

Figure 5

It may appear that the proposed model cannot accommodate either these results or the other discriminatory facts about blindsight subjects. For if the relevant portion of the grouped array is

[12] Marcel's forthcoming work here is described by Weiskrantz (1990). The first person to utilize this strategy was Torjussen (1978).

tion of the spatial attention system on the grouped array. Introspection in such cases is a process that takes visual experiences as inputs and yields beliefs about those experiences as outputs. So, introspective awareness is quite distinct from spatial attention. What spatial attention does is to contribute directly to visual experience or consciousness of external objects and their features, thereby determining in part the inputs to the process of introspection. It is not itself a component of that process. So, while it is true that blindsight subjects are not introspectively aware of undergoing visual experiences with respect to their scotoma, the reason for this is not that there is some defect in the process of introspection itself but rather that there are no visual *experiences* as such in these cases, and hence no inputs to the process of introspection.

empty then there is no information available there for processing by the object recognition system or the spatial attention system.

This response ignores the fact that there is a second major subcortical pathway from the eyes to the brain which is intact in blindsight subjects, and which does not feed into the grouped array. This pathway projects from the retina to the superior colliculus, and continues through the pulvinar to various parts of the cortex including both the parietal lobe and area V4 in the ventral system. It is known as the tecto-pulvinar pathway.[13]

Research with golden hamsters (by Schneider, 1969) suggests that one important role played by the tecto-pulvinar pathway is to orient the eyes reflexively towards a novel stimulus. It has been hypothesized that this pathway supports a wholly stimulus-based attention shifting system whose purpose is to move the eyes appropriately (see Kosslyn and Koenig, 1992). In blindsight subjects, then, correct eye movements in the blind field may be traced to the proper functioning of this system.

A further hypothesis, due to Lawrence Weiskrantz (1986), is that blindsight subjects can use the tecto-pulvinar pathway to extract information about features like movement, orientation, and position with respect to stimuli in the blind field. This capacity underlies the accurate guesses blindsight subjects make (in response to instructions).[14] It also appears that the shape recognition part of the object recognition system has access to information in this pathway. In Marcel's experiment cited above, such information is not sufficent on its own to trigger any shape identification. However, when combined with information about shape in the sighted field derived from processing of the contents of the filled portion of the grouped array, it gives rise to the phenomenon I described earlier.

There are many questions that remain here. But I cannot pursue them further in the present paper. Instead, I want now to take up again the Absent Qualia Hypothesis and some related philosophical issues.

III

I suggested in the last section that in blindsight the portion of the grouped array corresponding to the blind field is empty. As a result, there is no processing of this portion either by the object

---

[13] There are further subcortical pathways from the eyes to the brain. See here Weiskrantz (1990).

[14] So, it is a serious mistake to assume a priori, as McGinn (1991, pp. 111–112) does that there is a common underlying causal structure at play in both sight and blindsight. If Weiskrantz's hypothesis is correct, the mechanisms responsible for the discriminations made in the two cases have little in common.

recognition system or by the spatial attention system. It follows that there are important underlying functional differences between blindsight subjects and normally sighted people. These differences manifest themselves in behavioral differences, in, for example, the need for instructions to guess or the failure to draw shapes presented only to the blind field.[15] So, the phenomenon of blindsight clearly does *not* supply us with an example from real life that may be used to support, or partially illustrate, the Absent Qualia Hypothesis.[16] Let us turn next to some more general observations that may be brought to bear on the Hypothesis.

The four visual impairments I have discussed—apperceptive agnosia, dorsal simultanagnosia, ventral simultanagnosia, and blindsight—are all impairments in which normal visual experience is interrupted or altered in various ways. These impairments arise, according to the model I have sketched, because some component of the cognitive architecture underlying normal visual experience is not functioning properly. In the case of apperceptive agnosics, there is a defect in the grouping processes. As a result, there typically do not look to be whole shapes present, but there remains normal phenomenal awareness of features in purely local regions of the visual field.[17] For dorsal simultanagnosics, the defect is an attentional one. These subjects have normal visual experience with respect to a very limited portion of the field, but no consciousness at all with respect to the remainder. For blindsight subjects, there is also no consciousness with respect to part of the field, but the

---

[15] It should also be noted that blindsight subjects typically do not believe what they say about the blind field—their responses are forced guesses. This is a further respect in which they differ from normally sighted subjects. One philosopher who completely ignores this difference in his discussion of blindsight is John Heil (1983).

It does not help, I might add, to say, as Heil does, that blindsight subjects have unconscious beliefs with respect to the blind field. (Another philosopher who takes this view is Hugh Mellor (1977).) This locates the problem in the wrong place: there is nothing wrong with the mechanism of introspective awareness in such subjects. See here note 11 above.

Do blindsight subjects *see* the features with respect to which they make accurate guesses? In my view, the concept of seeing is a prototype concept. Blindsight is clearly not a prototypical case of seeing. Still it may be sufficiently similar to prototypical cases to count as a peripheral example. This seems to me an empirical matter. See here Tye (1992).

[16] Here I am in agreement with Dennett (1991).

[17] It is sometimes suggested that what it is like for apperceptive agnosics is similar to what it would be like for normally sighted people were they to don 'peppery' masks (that is, mask with many tiny apertures).

impairment this time concerns the grouped array and the processes that fill it. Finally, for ventral simultanagnosics, there is slowed visual awareness of more complicated shapes and multiple objects.

One reasonable hypothesis, then, is that the model I have presented reveals, in broad outline, the cognitive architecture responsible for normal human visual experience. Now, in general in cognitive psychology, the relationship between the phenomenon modelled and the phenomena modelling it is one of realization. A model of image generation, for example, presents an architecture that realizes the process of image generation in certain creatures, namely human beings. In this respect, cognitive psychology is just like other branches of science. For the relation of realization is the scientific glue that typically attaches higher level types (states, conditions, processes) to their lower level counterparts (see Tye, 1992). So, one proposal worth taking very seriously, I suggest, is that, in the standard case, visual experience is *realized* in human beings by the action of three key elements operating at all representational levels in the normal way: (i) a grouped array that has been properly filled by processes operating on information from the eyes, and that represents the surfaces visible from the relevant point of view together with their local features; (ii) a spatial attention system operating on the grouped array; and (iii) an object (including shape) recognition system operating in parallel with the spatial attention system on the grouped array. This proposal, as I shall now show, has implications for the Absent Qualia Hypothesis.

The realization relation is at least in part one of determination: the lower level property or type synchronically fixes the higher level one (so that the tokening of the former at any time t necessitates the tokening of the latter at t but not conversely). The relevant notion of necessity here is both nomological and strict (that is, without any *ceteris paribus* qualifications). Under the present proposal, then, any creature or machine, that has the systems specified in conditions (i)–(iii) above and operating (at all representational levels) in the way such systems operate in normal humans, *necessarily* has visual experiences. It follows that such a creature or machine cannot be wholly without experiences.

If we are to bring this result to bear on the Absent Qualia Hypothesis, we need to consider what it is for a creature to be functionally exactly like us. Suppose, to begin with, we adopt the following purely causal account : a creature is a human functional isomorph if, and only if, it has a system of inner states that causally interact with one another and with certain physical inputs and outputs just as our mental states do. Then it follows that the

Absent Qualia Hypothesis is false, given the further assumption that the presence of the appropriate causal interactions is sufficient for the tokening of the various representational states posited in the proposed model. Assumptions of this sort are widely accepted by philosophers, and they are also typically accepted by advocates of the Absent Qualia Hypothesis (see, for example, Block, 1990). So, I suggest that, on the proposal I have made, the Absent Qualia Hypothesis (interpreted causally) is seriously threatened.[18]

Suppose alternatively that we take a creature to be a human functional isomorph if, and only if, it is subject to a system of states and processes that are identical in their teleofunctional roles to those underlying normal human mentality at every psychological level. Then, again it seems to me that the present proposal creates trouble for the Absent Qualia Hypothesis. Let me explain.

The purpose of the human visual system is to enable us to make accurate discriminations with respect to distal objects on the basis of information contained in the light reaching our eyes. The grouped array contributes to this purpose, I maintain, by serving another one, namely that of representing information about features of the visible surfaces regardless of the objects to which the surfaces belong. So, if the cognitive architecture of human vision conforms to Farah's model, any full-fledged teleofunctional human isomorph will automatically be subject to states that play the representational roles of states of the grouped array. More generally, any such isomorph will certainly meet the conditions specified earlier for realizing visual experience in human beings.[19] So, any creature that is, in this sense, functionally identical with us will *have* to be subject to visual experiences.

In closing this section, I should note that the stronger conclusions I have reached here about the Absent Qualia Hypothesis assume that the Hypothesis is interpreted as asserting that it is *nomically* possible for there to be a creature or machine that is functionally equivalent to normal human beings but that lacks any feeling or experience. Under this interpretation, the only relevant

---

[18] What is required to alleviate the threat is an argument that mental representation is *not* causally determined in the appropriate ways. For one such argument, focussing on the case of *wide* causal determination, see Tye (forthcoming).

[19] I am supposing here that, whatever the level of decomposition, all the states and processes posited in psychological theories or models of the same general sort as Farah's have their own teleofunctional roles (relative to the relevant organisms). States and processes at higher levels play their roles in virtue of being decomposable into lower-level states and processes that also have teleofunctional characterizations.

possible worlds, as far as the Hypothesis is concerned, are ones in which *our* laws of nature obtain. If it is held that there are metaphysically possible worlds which are nomically impossible, then the argument I have presented leaves the Hypothesis untouched. For, as I noted earlier, the kind of necessity appropriate to the realization relation is nomological.

The conclusions I have reached about the nomic impossibility of absent experience also rest upon another hypothesis I do not claim to have established, even given that the model used to explain the earlier impairments is along the right lines. The hypothesis, of course, is that normal visual experience in humans is *realized* by the specified cognitive structures. I suggested earlier that this hypothesis is worth taking very seriously. But it is not the only possibility. For, it is compatible with my earlier remarks on how blindsight and the other impairments interrupt visual experience that the proper operation of the relevant cognitive systems is only necessary for normal visual experience in human beings without being sufficient. One alternative conjecture, then, is that visual experience of the sort found in normally sighted human-beings is realized by the joint action of the various components of the specified cognitive architecture *and* a certain neurophysiology.[20] On this view, while the cognitive components fix or determine the representational contents of the experiences, they do not by themselves generate any phenomenology. It is only in combination with the right hardware that states with the phenomenal features of human visual experiences are produced. So, in systems that have the architecture but lack our neurophysiology, it remains an open question whether or not they have any visual *consciousness*.

The question of how to decide between these two alternative proposals is a large one, which I cannot take up here. Instead, in the final section, I want to consider briefly whether either proposal goes any way towards removing the alleged mystery of consciousness.

IV

It seems clear that there is no single concept, or problem, of consciousness. One issue that has vexed many philosophers, and that is sometimes taken to be the most pressing problem of consciousness, is that of explaining how neural states give rise to phenome-

---

[20] I cannot take up here the question of whether the cognitive architecture is itself wholly neurally realized. The central issue is whether the representational contents of components of the architecture (e.g., the grouped array) are wide or narrow. See here Tye (forthcoming).

nal experiences and feelings. Colin McGinn (1991, p. 1) puts the problem this way:

> How is it possible for conscious states to depend upon brain states? How can technicolor phenomenology arise from soggy grey matter? What makes the bodily organ we call the brain so radically different from other bodily organs, say the kidneys— body parts without a trace of consciousness? How could the aggregation of millions of individually insentient neurons generate subjective awareness?

McGinn has concluded that we cannot answer these questions, that for us consciousness must remain an unfathomable mystery.

If the first proposal made in the last section is correct, however, then we do have answers to these questions at least in very broad outline, provided that their scope is restricted to the case of normal visual experience. Here conscious states depend on brain states in virtue of the brain states supporting the specified cognitive architecture. One striking difference between the brain and the other bodily organs is the fact that it alone supports this architecture. Millions of insentient neurons generate subjective awareness of the sort typically found in vision by co-operatively interacting so as to produce the requisite systems and operations.[21]

No doubt it will be replied that the mystery associated with visual consciousness has not really been removed on this proposal, only transferred elsewhere. For the question now arises as to how it is that the described cognitive structures and operations *themselves* produce visual experience or awareness. How is it that *these* states generate 'technicolor phenomenology'?

Regrettably, I do not have a fully satisfying answer to this question. But I think I can locate just where the puzzle presently lies. Let me begin by trying to say something illuminating about the more restricted question of how phenomenal variations *within* visual experiences are generated on my first proposal. I have argued elsewhere (Tye, 1991a; Tye, forthcoming) that two token visual experiences with the same representational content have the same phenomenal character, and that two token visual experiences with the same phenomenal character have the same representa-

---

[21] If one takes the view that what goes on inside the head does not alone suffice for the proposed cognitive architecture, since the architecture is representational, then the claims made in the last three sentences will need to be qualified by assertions concerning the environment and our causal interactions with it. This is not my own view (see Tye, forthcoming).

tional content (in so far as that content pertains to directly visible properties, e.g., colour and shape).[22] If this is correct, then an explanation can be given of what it is about the specified cognitive architecture that is responsible for differences in phenomenal character obtaining between visual experiences in terms of representational differences obtaining between certain portions of the grouped array upon which the spatial attention system is focussed and also (where appropriate) between certain active states in the shape recognition system.

Now it is often supposed that there is a *general* kind of consciousness which is essential to perceptual experiences and bodily sensations (phenomenal consciousness). This requires a little explanation before we proceed any further with the question of how visual experience or awareness is generated.

To have a pain is to feel a pain, and to feel a pain is to be conscious of pain. Similarly to seem to see something is to undergo a visual experience, and to undergo a visual experience is to be conscious of something visually. Consciousness, then, seems *intrinsic* to perceptual experiences and bodily sensations in a way in which it is not to belief and desire, for example. The latter states may or may not be conscious. They become conscious via the formation of second-order beliefs, or so it seems reasonable to suppose. I am aware of my belief that philosophy is hard, say, just in case I believe that I have the belief that philosophy is hard. But intuitively second-order belief is not intrinsic to the having of perceptual experiences and bodily sensations. Arguably, a simple creature could have a sensation, and in so doing have it consciously, without even having any first-order beliefs. At any rate, nothing in our concept of a sensation seems to rule out this possibility.

We are led, then, to distinguish a belief-laden kind of consciousness and another more primitive kind of consciousness, which is tied to feeling and experience.[23] The latter type of consciousness goes with talk of 'what it is like'. It is also associated with the inverted spectrum hypothesis and, as we have seen, the absent qualia hypothesis, although it does not presuppose that

---

[22] Other philosophers who hold a view of this sort (and who have influenced my own thinking) are Mark DeBellis (1991, and forthcoming) and Gilbert Harman (1990).

[23] Another possibility is that there are two general types of phenomenal consciousness, one for perceptual experiences and the other for bodily sensations. I discuss this issue in my 'Does pain lie within the domain of cognitive psychology?' (in preparation).

either of these hypotheses is true. Moreover, it seems transparent to introspective awareness.[24]

I very much doubt that the concept of phenomenal consciousness can be explained further by means of a reductive analysis. But this is, of course, no cause for special concern. Concepts generally lack reductive analyses. What I have tried to do above is to clarify the concept without analysing it.

Now since phenomenal consciousness is always consciousness of something or other, we might plausibly claim that when it is supplemented by the right representational contents (specifically contents involving the appropriate secondary qualities), it produces states with the phenomenal characters of the different species of perceptual experience. Within the context of the first proposal from Section III, then, this idea, in turn, naturally leads to the view that part of the phenomenal character of a given visual experience is due to its involving the generic intentional state type, phenomenal consciousness, and part due to aspects of its representational content. So, what really remains unexplained on the first proposal (with the above development), is how phenomenal consciousness is generated by the specified cognitive architecture.

Let me turn briefly to the alternative proposal I made at the end of the last section. The suggestion was that the phenomenal character of visual experiences is tied both to the cognitive architecture and to the neurophysiology. This suggestion can be developed further in a way that is compatible with my remarks about representational content and phenomenal character. In this case, we can suppose that part of the phenomenal character of a given visual experience has a non-representational neural realization, namely the generic state type, phenomenal consciousness, and part is realized by the appropriate higher level representational states and operations.

[24] This point is the one G. E. Moore (1922) was making when he characterized the sensation of blue as diaphonous. Focus your attention on a square that has been painted blue. Intuitively, you are directly aware of blueness and squareness as out there in the world, as features of an external surface. Now shift your gaze inward, and try to become aware of your experience, apart from its objects. The task seems impossible : ones awareness seems always to slip through the experience to its specific external intentional content—to the fact that it represents something outside as being blue and square. Similar observations apply in the case of pain. Focus your attention on some pain you are feeling. Now try to switch your awareness to the general activity of feeling which is integral to it. Again what one seems to end up attending to is simply the pain itself, the object of feeling.

The question which remains unanswered, of course, on this view, is, that of how the generic type, phenomenal consciousness, is itself generated by neural state types.[25] So, on both the pure non-neural proposal and on the second hybrid one, there is, I grant, a significant gap in our understanding of the production of visual experience.

The situation we find ourselves in here with respect to the generation of phenomenal consciousness contrasts markedly with the sort of understanding we have achieved in science with respect to certain other realizations. Take, for example, the realization of temperature in a gas by mean molecular kinetic energy.[26] Or consider the realization of elasticity in a rubber band by a certain molecular structure. In both these instances, an explanatory account *is* available of how the lower level properties generate the properties they realize which makes the generational link between the properties fully intelligible. Thus, in the case of elasticity, once we learn that the underlying molecular structure consists of long, partly coiled chain molecules that are highly flexible and mobile, we are in a position to appreciate that they can alter their arrangements and extensions in space in response to the application of force, thereby allowing the band to stretch. We can also understand in outline how it is that the band returns to its original state when the force is removed, once we are told further that pairs of segments in the long chain molecules, roughly one out of every hundred, are cross-linked in a network structure, thereby preventing the chains from sliding irreversibly by one another, and that the structure as

[25] Crick and Koch (1990) have hypothesized that neuronal oscillations in the 40 MHz range underlie phenomenal consciousness. This is an intriguing proposal, but even if true, without further development, it still does not put the matter fully to rest. How exactly does 40 MHz do the trick? Why isn't 30 MHz enough or 40 MHz too little? We currently have no adequate answers to these questions. It is also worth observing that the Crick-Koch hypothesis does not automatically favour the second proposal concerning phenomenal consciousness over the first non-neural one. For it could be that, in the case of vision, the 40 MHz oscillation generates a cognitive process in the specified architecture (for example, the operation of the spatial attention system on the grouped array) which, in turn, generates phenomenal consciousness.

[26] Some philosophers have supposed that the relationship here is one of identity. This is clearly mistaken, however. In a solid, temperature is something different, since the molecules are confined to certain restricted periodic motions. In a plasma, there are no constituent molecules, but there is temperature. Finally, in a vacuum, there is 'blackbody' temperature in the distribution of electromagnetic waves, although, there is certainly no molecular kinetic energy. See here Churchland (1988).

a whole has a tendency to increase its entropy towards the maximum value it had in its undeformed state.[27]

In the case of mean molecular kinetic energy, the connection with temperature is effected via pressure and volume. Boyle's Law informs us that for an ideal gas, temperature is a function of the product of pressure and volume. According to the kinetic theory of gases, mean molecular energy is likewise a function of the product of gas pressure and volume. A certain molecular energy E generates a certain temperature T, then, for a given sample of gas, since E is the energy that corresponds to T for the relevant volume and pressure.

No comparable account is currently available for the realization of phenomenal consciousness on either of the two proposals I have considered. So here, it seems evident, we do not now have full understanding. It would be highly premature, however, to conclude that such understanding will necessarily *always* escape us, that there is here a mystery which we cannot solve. Only fools rush in where scientists have yet fully to tread.[28]

[27] Stretching out the chains decreases their entropy.

[28] I am indebted to Tony Marcel and Alex Rosenberg for helpful discussion, and to David Chalmers for written comments.

References

Block, N. 1980, 'Troubles with functionalism', in N. Block (ed.), *Readings in the Philosophy of Psychology*, Volume 1. Cambridge, Mass.: Harvard University Press.

Block, N. and Fodor, J. 1980. 'What psychological states are not', in N. Block (ed.) *Readings in the Philosophy of Psychology*, Volume 1. Cambridge, Mass.: Harvard University Press.

Block, N. 1990 'Inverted earth' in J. Tomberlin (ed.), *Philosophical Perspectives*, Volume 4. Atascadero, CA: Ridgeview Publishing Company.

Campbell, K. 1980. *Body and Mind*. Notre Dame: University of Notre Dame Press.

Churchland, P. 1988. *Matter and Consciousness*. Cambridge, Mass.: The MIT Press.

Crick, F. and Koch, C. 1990. 'Toward a neurobiological theory of consciousness', *Seminars in the Neurosciences*, **2**, 263–275.

DeBellis, M. 1991. 'The representational content of musical experience', *Philosophy and Phenomenolgical Research*, **51**, 303–324.

DeBellis, M. forthcoming. *Music and Conceptualization*. Cambridge University Press.

Dennett, D. 1991. *Consciousness Explained*. Little Brown.

Efron, R. 1968. 'What is perception?' *Boston Studies in Philosophy of Science* **4**, 159.

Farah, M. 1991. Visual Agnosia. Cambridge, Mass.: The MIT Press.

Godwin-Austen, R. 1965. 'A case of visual disorientation', *Journal of Neurology, Neurosurgery and Psychiatry* **28**, 453–458.

Harman, G. 1990. 'The intrinsic qualities of experience', in J. Tomberlin (ed.), *Philosophical Perspectives*, Volume 4, Atascadero, CA: Ridgeview Publishing Company.

Heil, J. 1983. *Perception and Cognition*. University of California Press.

Hecaen, H. and Ajuriaguerra, J. 1974 'Agnosie visuelle pour les objets inanimes par lesion unilaterale gauche', *Revue Neurologique*, **12**, 447–464.

Kosslyn, S. and Koenig, O. 1992. *Wet Minds*. New York: The Free Press.

Landis, T., Graves, R., Benson, F., Hebben, N. 1982. 'Visual recognition through kinaesthetic mediation', *Psychological Medicine*, **12**, 515–531.

Lycan, W. 1987. *Consciousness*. Cambridge, Mass.: The MIT Press.

Marr, D. 1982. *Vision*. San Francisco: W. H. Freeman.

McGinn, C. 1991. *The Problem of Consciousness*. Oxford: Blackwells.

Mellor, H. 1977 'Conscious belief', *Proceedings of the Aristotelian Society*, **68**, 87–101.

Moore, G. E. 1922. *Philosophical Studies*. London: Routledge and Kegan Paul.

Nagel, T. 1980. 'What is it like to be a bat?' in N. Block (ed.) *Readings in the Philosophy of Psychology*, Volume 1, Cambridge, Mass.: Harvard University Press.

Schneider, G. 1969. 'Two visual systems', *Science*, **163**, 895–902.

Torjussen, T. 1978. 'Visual processing in cortically blind hemifields', *Neuropsychologia* **16**, 15–21.

Tye, M. 1986. 'The subjective qualities of experience', *Mind*, **95**, 1–17.

Tye, M. 1991a. 'Visual qualia and visual content', in T. Crane (ed.), *The Contents of Experience: Essays on Perception*. Cambridge: Cambridge University Press.

Tye, M. 1991b. *The Imagery Debate*. Cambridge, Mass: The MIT Press.

Tye, M. 1992. 'Naturalism and the mental', *Mind*, **101**, 421–441.

Tye, M. forthcoming. 'Qualia, content and the inverted spectrum', *Nous*.

Tyler, H. 1968. 'Abnormalities of perception with defective eye movements (Blaint's syndrome)', *Cortex*, **3**, 154–171.

Ungerleider, L. and Mishkin, M. 'Two cortical visual systems', in D. Ingle, M. Goodale, and R. Mansfield (ed.), *Analysis of Visual Behavior*. Cambridge, Mass.: The MIT Press.

Weiskrantz, L. 1986. *Blindsight : A Case Study and its Implications*. New York: Oxford University Press.

Weiskrantz, L. 1990. 'Outlooks for blindsight : explicit methodologies for implicit processes', *Proceedings of the Royal Society London*, **239**, 247–278.

Do Your Concepts Develop?*

ANDREW WOODFIELD

'Psychological structures may be shown to grow and differentiate throughout life. Correspondingly, the brain has a much more lengthy and involved development than any other mechanism of the body. We know little yet of how this uniquely complex process is determined, but it is certain that the principles of embryogenesis apply in all growth, including psychological growth, and not just to the morphogenesis of the body of the embryo.'
Colwyn B. Trevarthen (1973), 'Behavioral Embryology' (p. 89)

I. Representations That Develop Within The Individual

Though *development* is fundamentally a biological notion, it is fruitfully employed in many other branches of science. Psychology is certainly an area in which developmental questions arise. Everyone agrees that the child's mind develops. However, not everyone agrees that the child's *concepts* develop. Some philosophers would say that although there are analogies between mental growth and bodily growth, the analogy ceases to be fruitful at the level of concepts, because concepts have intentional contents, and their contents cannot change. The aim of this paper is examine the pros and cons of the proposition that a person's concepts can develop.

As usual in these matters, the thesis that concepts develop admits of many interpretations. Let me start by explaining how the thesis will be construed in this paper. The following four points will serve to define a more precise target-thesis which we may then go on to criticize. The thesis to be targeted is by no means a straw man. It is a doctrine to which many developmental psychologists would assent.

(i) The thesis is not just that a child's *repertoire* of concepts grows over time. It says something about the child's concepts taken one by one. It says that any concept that the subject possess-

*Thanks to Kent Bach, Marcos Barbosa de Oliveira, Andrew Brennan, Laurence Goldstein, Stephan Körner and Adam Morton for comments on an earlier version. Steve Stich and other participants at the Birmingham conference helped by asking searching questions. I also had the benefit of discussing these issues with John McShane in the summer of 1992, shortly before his tragic death.

es can change some of its properties while retaining its individual identity. This thesis is stronger than the claim that a child adds new concepts to his previous network. To test the thesis, a psychologist would have to track particular nodes of the network over time. This would, of course, involve longtitudinal study of the child whose network it is.

It may be that a child's concept-network is so constituted that if any concept within it were to undergo a certain type of qualitative change, this would inevitably have repercussions elsewhere in the network. But if a whole set of concepts can change, it has to be possible for a single concept to undergo a change.

(ii) Proponents of the thesis use descriptive phrases like 'Susie's concept of *cats*', and the schematic 'S's concept of K', intending to refer to a *personal possession*. A personal concept is identified partly by reference to its owner. If Susie has one concept of *milk* and Tommy also has one concept of *milk*, there are two distinct psychological particulars of the type, *concept of milk*. That they are of the same type does not imply they are exactly similar. One of the research goals of developmental psychology is to discover whether there are similarities between children in a given cohort with respect to the concepts that they have.

Speakers sometimes use descriptions like 'the concept of *milk*' intending to refer to a publicly shared concept abstracted from individual possessors. Public concepts are in a different ontological category from the psychological structures that concern us here. The thesis that a personal concept can change during its owner's lifetime must be sharply separated from the claim that a public concept can change over time. Questions like 'Has the concept of *masculinity* altered in the last 20 years?', or 'Did the concept of *force* alter as a result of Newton?', are *irrelevant* to developmental psychology, at least in the pure case. A pure case would be a person who formed and developed her own concept of K during an era when the public concept of K remained static. Of course, if a child's formative years coincide with a period of rapid linguistic and cultural change, the community's changing standards may influence her personal intellectual development. But that is an impure case.

(iii) Proponents of the target thesis take a personal concept to be a mental representation. Nearly all modern textbooks in developmental psychology seem to agree on this.[1]

---

[1] An example from a recent textbook: 'Concepts are the products of categorization. The term 'concept' refers to a mental representation that determines how entities are related.' (McShane 1991, p. 124).

This postulate conflicts with the view that a concept is an abstract entity, a view associated with the logician Frege. It marks a theoretical stance which Frege condemned as 'psychologism'. But psychologists don't care about being psychologistic; they think that they are *justified*. They reason thus: when a person *grasps* a Fregean concept, the person forms a representation in his or her own mind. There is no other way of doing it. Therefore: (a) personal mental representations exist, (b) they are legitimate objects of study by psychologists (though perhaps not by logicians). Frege's doctrines about concepts and thoughts leave open the possibility of the existence of such mental representations, even though he reserves the word 'concept' for something other than a mental representation.[2]

Because most contemporary cognitive psychologists believe the mind is realized in the brain as software is realized in hardware, there is wide agreement that concepts, construed as mental representations, are *internal* representations. The physicalist doctrine that every concept possessed by S is embodied in some part of S's neural circuitry will henceforth be called the *IRTC* (short for 'Internal Representation Theory of Concepts').

Most IRTC people hold that the mental representations used in higher thought-processes are functionally different from percepts and images, as well as being quite different from subpersonal (or 'subdoxastic') representations. However, there are various views within IRTC, some competing, some complementary, about the precise form and functional structure characteristic of a concept. It will not be within the scope of this paper to compare or evaluate these alternatives.

(iv) The changes that constitute *development*, in the relevant sense, are changes in the *semantic content* of a concept. No opinion is expressed about whether a concept develops in non-semantic ways. We shall focus upon kind-concepts, and the changes will be hypothesized changes of extension and/or intension.

Psychologists think that a young child can possess a kind-concept that is not fully developed. For example, McShane (1991, p. 153), discussing children's over-overcautiousness in the use of words, says 'the fact that words are not always extended to include the peripheral instances of a concept suggests that the concept

---

[2] Cf. Macnamara 1986, Preface, p. X: 'I saw that even if we take the most extreme antipsychologistic position, even if we take the Platonist view that logical structures exist outside the mind in a realm beyond time and space, these structures must be realized in our minds somehow if we are to apply them in our thinking.'

itself may not be fully developed but may instead be concentrated around prototypical exemplars'.

Yet the idea that a concept can change its extension (or its intension) is problematic. Some philosophers would deny that a concept can become more fully developed by altering its extension.[3] They argue that the hypothesis is incoherent, because the extension of a given concept individuates the concept. Since the supposed change is logically impossible, there can be no such developmental process.

This *a priori* dismissal appears high-handed to psychologists, and they generally ignore it.[4] Yet the challenge must be answered; it cannot be swept under the carpet. The debate will be joined in section III, after we have placed the target-thesis in a biological context. To readers who are psychologists, I issue a word of warning. The issue in this debate is fundamentally a question of *ontology*. As such, the debate will strike some people as arcane, even Scholastic. Nevertheless, I am convinced that the ontological issue —concerning the existence and individuation of personal concepts —needs to be urgently addressed, in order that the foundations of the theory of conceptual development be made secure.

II. Influences From Embryology

In this section I introduce a few of the notions from developmental biology which have found their way into psychology. Developmental psychology is a relatively young science. Its pioneers were willing to borrow from more established disciplines, and embryology supplied them with a paradigm. It is understandable that fledgling sciences should look to more advanced sciences for inspiration. In this case, there was also a particular historical reason. Jean Piaget was trained in embryology before he became a 'genetic epistemologist'. In his (translated) autobiography, he says, 'my aim of discovering a sort of embryology of intelligence . . . fit (*sic*) in with my biological training' (Piaget 1973, p. 120). Piaget's personal influence upon the discipline has been enormous. In retrospect, perhaps it was unfortunate that embryology should have been such an important source of theories and terminology. For it

[3] Such a view is implicit in Fodor's view of concept-learning. See Fodor (1975, 1980, 1981).

[4] Carey (1985) and Keil (1989), for instance, investigate conceptual development experimentally without worrying overmuch about the niceties of concept-individuation.

was, until recently, a backward and confused branch of biology. Foetal development, still poorly understood, presents one of the greatest intellectual challenges for the next century.[5]

Consider first the notion of a *developmental process*. Where there is development, there is something that develops. Developing can be split into two phases: a *coming-to-be* phase and a *subsequent modification* phase. In the latter phase, there has to be a persisting entity (a whole organism, an organ, or a part) which is the subject of changes. In tracing the history of such an entity, one assumes principles of identity across time. For a physical organ, these will comprise principles specific to the kind of organ it is, plus a principle of spatio-temporal continuity.[6]

Anyone who assumes that a particular at time t_2 is the same individual as a particular at t_1 ought to be able to supply a 'covering sortal' (Wiggins 1980). A covering sortal is a count noun naming a type of thing T such that the earlier particular is a T and the later particular is a T. Only if there is a covering sortal can one sensibly claim that the former is the same individual as the latter, according to Wiggins, because the principles that determine diachronic sameness derive in part from the nature of the type T.[7]

Given that a certain T thing exists at t_1 and subsequently develops, the stages of the developmental process are unified as stages of the *same* process partly by virtue of the fact that they all involve the same T. A *developmental explanation* would identify the causes of the changes undergone by the individual T thing. Such causes might be endogenous or environmental. The whole story would show how mixtures of internal and external causes at each stage jointly produced the next stage.[8]

Before the T thing can get modified, it has to have come into being. The first phase of development is formation. Here, too, we need a covering-sortal, because *formation* is the formation of something of a specifiable kind. The sortal determines whether something put up as a candidate counts as a member of the kind. Suppose that no T thing existed at time t_1 in a certain spatial

[5] Compare the remarks in Woodger 1929, p. 352.

[6] But see Brennan (1988, pp. 37–51), who discusses problems with the notion of continuity and countenances the possibility of entities (e.g. mental entities) whose histories are discontinuous.

[7] Brennan (ibid.) considers the claim that an entity can persist even if there is no covering sortal (apart from dummy-sortals like 'thing'). But it remains true that in real examples of biological development, covering sortals are expected.

[8] This view of developmental explanation is endorsed by Sober (1984) pp. 147–155, who contrast it with selectional explanation.

region of a body, and later, at t_2, a T thing is found there. Other explanations of the presence of the T being ruled out, we conclude that it is the product of development. Previously existing things interacted in such a way as to create a new thing. Some of the antecedents might have become *ingredients* of the newly created T. There might have been one antecedent thing, not itself a T, which played a sufficiently pivotal role to warrant our saying that it *turned into* a T. For example, a particular cluster of cells present in an embryo at t_1 might be transformed into something identifiable at t_2 as an *eye*. But in other cases no particular ingredient stands out as being 'the T-to-be', because none has a greater claim than any of the other ingredients.

The dividing point between the process of a T's formation and the phase of its subsequent modification is the moment of *coming to be*. In the case of an animal, birth is a conveniently salient moment. Yet we know that a baby's organs do not really come into existence at the moment of its birth, any more than the baby itself does. If we ask 'At what moment did this baby's right index finger first come into existence?', the embryologist has to say that there was no precise moment. The process was gradual. The conditions for being a right index finger are somewhat vague. For a period of several weeks it is indeterminate whether THIS portion of the foetus (the portion whose fate is to become a right index finger) is *already* a right index finger. Embryologists cannot locate a precise borderline between the 'formation' phase and the 'subsequent modification' phase, even though the conceptual distinction between the two phases seems valid.

Perhaps it is because of this natural blurring that the same term, 'developing', covers both phases. Embryologists officially study both the formation and the early life-history of organs. Likewise, developmental psychologists wish to study *both* concept-formation[9] and modifications in concepts that have already been formed. So the total development of S's concept of K comprises two successive

[9] If you are a psychologist, the choice between the terms 'forming' and 'acquiring' ought to be highly significant, for they have different ontological connotations. If someone 'acquires' a thing, it is not impossible that the thing existed before the person acquired it. All that may have happened is that the person entered into a new relation to it. By contrast, the 'forming' of a person's concept of K is the *coming into existence* in that person of something which meets the conditions for being of the type concept of K. If S *forms* a concept of K, that concept did not exist before. Once it is formed, S's relationship to it is a kind of inalienable ownership, like the relation between an organism and its heart. The concept is S's personal possession. I form my concepts, you form yours.

phases. The boundary between the phases is marked by the first moment at which S has truly attained a concept of K. Since this moment is hard to date, it might be better to think of the borderline as an interval whose beginning and end are fuzzy.

Piaget argues in many books that mental development is an *epigenetic* process. *Epigenesis* is a notion that he took over from embryology. Part of what he means is that the structure of the mind increases in complexity as a result of cycles of interaction between the child and his environment; mental growth is not merely a rearranging of cognitive structures that were present in the child at birth.

In embryology, 'epigenesis' is often defined in terms of a traditional contrast with *preformation*. Preformationism in its general form is the hypothesis that 'the egg at the time of fertilization already contains something corresponding to every feature that will eventually be present in the fully formed adult' (Waddington 1966, p. 15). Epigeneticism is merely the denial of this hypothesis. We now know that some structures found in adults (e.g. genes) are present in eggs, others are not. Microscopic livers, fingers, and frontal lobes are not. When early embryologists proposed that whole organs were preformed, their hypotheses were *bona fide*; but the claims turned out to be false. In the psychology of concepts, the analogue of preformationism is the hypothesis that all concepts are innate. Few people believe such an exaggerated claim. Many, however, believe that *some* concepts are innate. They think that concepts are internal structures, and that the postulation of a few such structures in neonates is empirically warranted.

Suppose that a certain child S has a concept which is present in S at birth and which persists. For the sake of an example which many will find plausible, let us suppose that it is a concept of *cause*. Even though it is innate, we can think of this concept's developmental life-history as comprising two phases, its 'formation' phase followed by its 'subsequent modification' phase, just as we can with any non-innate concept. The question 'How did that concept originate in S?' still requires a detailed scientific answer. There must be some story to tell about how it got formed. Part of the story will presumably make reference to instructions encoded in the genes, and it will show how those genes interacted with matter in S's embryo. This is the ontogenetic part of the story. To trace the story further back would presumably involve explaining why those genes were present in the nuclei of S's cells, and why they contained instructions for building a concept of *cause*. At this point, we switch from ontogenetic explanation to evolutionary explanation.

Innateness does not entail immutability. If S's concept of *cause* is like an innate organ, it might develop in various ways while continuing to be a concept of *cause*, in the same way that the right index finger of a baby grows bigger and stronger while continuing to be a right index finger. If there is anything objectionable in the thesis that a concept can change, the objection is *not* that change is incompatible with preformation.

Another embryological notion borrowed by developmental psychologists is *natural developmental trajectory*. A change does not qualify as a biological development unless it is a part of a sequence of changes exemplified in all normal organisms of the species at roughly the same age.[10] In fact, there are reliable diachronic generalizations about many physical processes. It is possible to construct a composite picture of the growth of a normal member of the species. For any change manifested by a real individual S at a given age, the criterion of its being a *developmental* change is whether the normal individual goes through the same sort of change around that age. If the change does qualify as a developmental change, the biologist can also determine whether S is retarded or advanced for its age in respect of that change.

Clearly there are many parameters which one may use to define a specific type of trajectory: the salient stages in it, the duration of each stage, the ordering of the stages, the speed of transition between stages, the age of the organism at each stage, the destination or endpoint, and so on.

According to Waddington (1966), a truly developmental trajectory will be to some degree 'homeorhetic'. By this he means that deviations from the normal track, induced by external interferences, are corrected. The normal individual gets back on track. Homeorhesis is the developmental analogue of homeostasis. Suppose the normal pathway goes from stage A to stage B to stage C. If the transition from A to B is delayed in S, the duration of stage B may be shortened so that the change from B to C takes place at the normal time. If the growth of a certain structure is accelerated for a while relative to other structures, it may slow down later, as if waiting for the others to catch up. A developmental trajectory is highly stable; forces conspire to keep it on track, almost as if there were an imperative for S to arrive at the proper destination at the proper time.[11]

[10] cf. Woodger (1929, p. 344): 'Although embryology is primarily concerned with the processes exhibited by the single individual organism as such it presupposes a race for obvious reasons. It works with the concept of 'normal' development, and this can only be reached if there is available a supply of embryos all manifesting much the same series of changes.'

[11] This feature has led some biologists to say that embryogenesis is a teleological process. But the meaning of 'teleological' is unclear. It is

The mental progress of a child is like a natural developmental trajectory in some respects. Piaget held that the normal child goes through certain psychological stages in a fixed order; for example, she lacks symbolic intelligence until she has passed through the concrete-operational stage. Certain general concepts emerge at roughly the same age in all children. Basic competences characteristic of a given age-group are manifested by all children of that age, irrespective of their culture or environment (within limits). There are even apparent examples of homeorhesis, as when a child who is backward at age 5 puts on a spurt at age 6, so that by age 7 she has caught up with her peers.

In sum, these embryological notions seem to have some value for psychology. If natural developments and trajectories are found at the level of the whole mind, then perhaps they are also to be found at the level of mental 'parts'. A commitment to this analogy lies behind the proposition that concepts develop. The analogy is deeply entrenched. For example, many psychologists say that a child's concepts are 'not fully fledged', and that an adult's concepts are 'mature', locutions which imply that conceptual growth moves to a natural destination—maturity—and then stops.

III. In-House Debate: Semantic Change Within a Single Concept

We now return to the problem of content-change. I shall explore it by staging a debate. One party, whom I shall call Preform, asserts that every concept has a static content. The opponent, Epigen, says that a concept can alter its content.

These two parties share a lot of common ground. Both accept that a particular concept in a network can be singled out and traced across time, that a concept is a personal possession, and that a concept is an internal representation. The debate takes place inside IRTC; neither party queries the basic assumptions of IRTC. Both agree, for example, that a child's set of personal con-

doubtful whether homeorhesis is sufficient proof that a process is objectively *goal-directed*. There is clearly an analogy with purposive journeying toward a destination, however, and this encourages the observer to *project* goal-directedness on to it. On the other hand, one can see reasons for saying that a teleological *function* is served by staying on the normal developmental track. There may well be a true natural selection story to explain why embryonic maturation processes are so resistant to interferences and individual contingencies. For more on the importance of not confusing different types of teleology, see Woodfield (1976).

cepts at one age is often somewhat different from her set of concepts at a later age. So they agree that there is change OF concepts. What the disputants disagree about is whether there can be change IN concepts, that is, change that occurs within a concept while that concept carries on existing.

According to McShane (1991), when a child underextends a word, this may be because the child's concept is *narrower in extension* than the adult concept expressed by the word. Let us take the case of Marie, a French girl. In early childhood she got to know various tabby and ginger cats, and learned to call them 'chat'. At age 3.0, Marie met a Siamese cat for the first time. On that occasion she was disinclined to call it 'chat'. Why? An explanation is offered as follows.

> *Marie aged 3.0 possessed an internal representation of cats, which included a specification of what a typical cat looks like. Her representation had been formed as a result of her experience of a limited range of cats. The Siamese did not fit Marie's prototype of a cat. Her concept's extension did not include it. Marie refrained from applying her concept to the Siamese, which is why she wouldn't apply the word. If we jump forward in time to Marie at age 4.0, we observe that she now happily calls this Siamese cat 'chat'. She seems to understand that it is a cat, albeit an unusual one. The developmentalist explanation is that Marie's concept used to be concentrated around prototypical exemplars. But her concept has developed. Now she applies it, correctly, to peripheral members of the category.*

This explanation may be challenged, on the grounds that it makes no sense to say that a concept widened its extension. Is it not an *essential feature* of a concept of cats that it has the class of cats as its extension? In everyday psychological interpretation we respect a 'Different Extension Implies Different Concept' Principle:

(P1) If concept type C1 differs in extension from concept type C2, then C1 and C2 are distinct types.

Principle (P1) states a necessary condition of type-identity. Appealing to this unassailable principle, an opponent of the proposition might try to argue that Marie's early concept must be numerically distinct from her later concept. His first move will be to argue that the developmentalist has *wrongly described Marie's situation*.

The story was that Marie aged 3.0 had a concept which covered tabbies and ginger cats but which excluded a Siamese, and that therefore its extension was not the whole class of cats but was rather a subclass, which we could call *shmats*. So, according to that story, it was not really a concept of cats. What she really had was a concept of *shmats*. By the age of 4.0, however, she has a concept which includes all cats; this one really is a concept of *cats*. The developmentalist claimed that the concept at 3.0 and the concept at 4.0 were one and the same. The anti-developmentalist says that they were numerically distinct because they belonged to distinct content-types. The anti-developmentalist accepts that the child developed, but he denies that a single concept developed.

At this point the developmentalist has to clarify his position. Both parties make the assumption that Marie's concept at 3.0 *denoted a narrow class*. Accepting Principle (P1), the developmentalist concedes that her concept at 3.0 was really a concept of *shmats*. Yet he goes on to point out that this concession does not undermine his thesis, because Principle (P1) does not rule out the possibility that a given concept-token might belong to different types at different times. Personal concepts, he will say, are real psychological individuals. When Marie's concept developed, it switched from being a token of *shmat* to being a token of *cat*, like a caterpillar metamorphosing into a butterfly. It has a real identity that isn't exhausted by the content it happens to have at a particular time. It is an entity about which counterfactual suppositions can be entertained. If Marie's life between 3.0. and 4.0 had run differently, the concept she had at 3.0 might not have turned into a concept of *cats* at 4.0 but might have become a concept of *zats*.

How can it be determined whether Marie's concept at 3.0 really is the same individual entity as her concept at 4.0? Consider the proposition: that boy in 1960 is the same individual as this man in 1990. Its truth or falsity can be determined because the boy was a human being and the man is a human being, and there are principles for tracing a human being across time. The term 'human being' is available as a covering sortal. Whenever we consider a diachronic identity question, we need a covering sortal 'T' such that we can ask 'Is the early T the same T as the later T?'

The developmentalist postulates an entity that went through a *phase* of being a concept of *shmats* when Marie was around 3 years old.[12] He

---

[12] Wiggins (1980) calls the term 'boy' a *phase sortal*, because it group together individuals of the same kind who occupy a given life-phase as *occupants of that phase in the life of the kind*. The term 'human being', in contrast, is a *substance sortal*: every human being is a life-long member of the category. Not every way of classifying individuals on the basis of their transient membership in a class involves classifying them under a phase sortal. For example, 'doctor' is not a phase sortal, nor is 'passenger in Concorde', and nor is 'concept of *shmats*'. Also, not every covering

thinks that its being a concept of *cats* is a phase too, a mature phase. But he hasn't yet revealed what kind of thing this changeable entity essentially and timelessly *is*. He must supply a covering sortal, and give principles for tracing identity under this sortal.

Supposing he were to find a suitable sortal 'T'. The discovery would profoundly affect his construal of the boundary-line between the 'coming-to-be' stage and the 'subsequent modification' stage. On the new construal, the first part of the development process would be the coming into existence of *that T*. The second part would be the modification of that T during its lifetime. All content changes would presumably occur within the second stage. For example, the process of becoming a concept of *cats* is a change that occurs to something already in existence which is not essentially or timelessly a concept of *cats*. There would no longer be any such process as the *formation* of Marie's concept of *cats*, since that would amount to the coming into being of an entity that was a (mature) concept of *cats* from the first moment of its existence.

Developmental psychologists make it their business to investigate the ages at which given concepts are formed. Hitherto we took this to be a matter of dating the 'births' of new concepts. It now seems we were misled. For the question 'When was Marie's concept of *cats* formed?' hides two separate questions.[13] One is a genuine question about origin: 'When did that T, which is now a (mature) concept of *cats*, first come into existence?' The answer is: 'Before Marie was aged 3.0.' The other question is not about origin, but is about the onset of a phase: 'When did that T turn into a concept of *cats*?'. The answer is: 'Some time between age 3.0 and age 4.0.'

Now that we are fully briefed about the background assumptions to which both disputants are committed, we are ready to eavesdrop on the debate between Epigen and Preform. Staging this debate seems to me to be a worthwhile philosophical exercise, because it illustrates the sorts of problems that arise when you take the thesis of concept-developmentalism absolutely literally. And, as I said before, the thesis is far from being a straw-man. Both

---

[13] A parallel case. You see an old newspaper photo of Elizabeth Taylor and Richard Burton on the day of their wedding. You ask 'How did that wife come into being?' You could either mean 'How did that person who is a wife come into being?', or mean 'How did that person come to marry Richard Burton?' Because of this ambiguity, the term 'wife' is not a good sortal under which to trace the identity of Elizabeth Taylor across time.

---

sortal needs to be a substance sortal, so long as it is a sortal that spans the period assumed by the diachronic identity question that is being asked.

sides in the dispute have actual adherents. The stance adopted by Preform closely resembles that of Jerry Fodor. Epigen, on the other hand, represents a position to which cognitive developmentalists on the whole subscribe, and which I, for several years, believed to be correct. By actually going through the moves and countermoves in this dialectic, we can, I hope, pinpoint a fundamental mistake.

Debate

EPIGEN: I propose that there exists in Marie a concept which goes through various phases during which it has different contents, and which ends up as her concept of *cats*. I shall introduce the term 'psi' as a rigid designator of this entity. For me, the main task is to specify what *kind* of thing psi is. I accept that I have the responsibility of explaining how to keep track of psi while it goes through these changes, and that this obliges me to find a suitable covering sortal.

PREFORM: I'll let you use the name 'psi', but your hypothesis that psi exists is merely a promissory note. I cannot see why you want to postulate a changing continuant to explain early word-learning, when there is a perfectly good alternative explanation available. The explanation goes roughly as follows.

When a child learns the meaning of a word, she successively tries out different hypotheses about what the word might mean. Marie evidently hypothesized at age 3.0 that 'chat' meant *shmat*, therein exercising her concept of *shmats*. That hypothesis got disconfirmed, so she tried another hypothesis. Probably she went through several intermediate steps before she hit on the correct hypothesis. Maybe at 3.6 she linked 'chat' to some other concept such as her concept of (let's say) *dats*, where the class of dats includes more cats but not all cats. Learning the meaning of a word is a matter of internal 'search' through a population of concepts that one already has. Marie tries to find the concept whose extension matches the extension of the word.[14]

Each concept-token is of a distinct content-type. And each one is semantically static. There is no need to say that any structure goes through semantic change; what happens is that S goes on an intellectual journey, activating first one structure, then the next. Developing is a process of becoming disposed to exercise some

[14] This view is advocated by Fodor (1975, 1980, 1981), and is widely accepted by psychologists. For example, Carey (1988, p. 174) says 'While children learn language from adults, they are not blank slates as regards their conceptual system. As they learn the terms of their language, they must map these onto the concepts they have available to them.'

concepts more readily than others. The conceptual structures themselves are fixed competences. Marie's trajectory through these structures is a temporally extended *performance* phenomenon.[15] *Figure 1* illustrates the true situation.

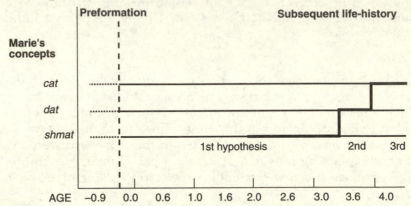

Figure 1 (*Note.* The bold line indicates which concept is actively associated with 'chat' at a given age).

EPIGEN: Your position may be clear, but it is empirically unbelievable. You have done a service to all developmentalists by providing a model of what to avoid.

You postulate a whole crowd of innate concepts. Because you are a believer in IRTC like me, you think each concept is realized in a neural structure in Marie's brain. As you know, the study of development includes the study of ontogenetic origin, as well as the study of change. If you are right that Marie is born with a large stock of concepts, then there must be an explanation of how they *came to be in Marie.* So you are committed to finding a multitude of origin explanations. Worse still, your story sets no upper limit on the number of concepts in Marie's head, since there is no limit on the number of possible concept-types with slightly different extensions which she might need tokens of, if she is to master the French language.

In claiming that these concepts are all innate, you hope to shift the problem of origin from psychology onto biology.[16]

[15] Thus Fodor (1980, p151): 'a theory of the conceptual plasticity of organisms must be a theory of how the environment selects among the innately specified concepts. *It is not a theory of how you acquire concepts, but a theory of how the environment determines which parts of the conceptual mechanism in principle available to you are in fact exploited.*'

[16] Fodor does just this: 'It looks as though the innate structure of the mind is going to be very rich indeed according to the present proposal. Our ethology promises to be quite interesting even if our developmental psychology turns out to be a little dull.' (Fodor 1981, pp. 315-6).

But you will not receive any support from evolutionary biologists. Leave aside the fact that there aren't enough distinct neurons in the brain to encode the potential infinities of concepts that you postulate. The main consideration, from an evolutionary point of view, is that Nature would not have been so wasteful as to provide them all in advance. The vast majority of these concepts will be completely useless to their possessor, because they will never be exercised. Of those that do get employed in the formulation of hypotheses, most will enjoy only fifteen minutes of stardom until their hypotheses are proved wrong, and then they are left to rot. So the huge set of preformed concepts that you require could never have evolved by natural selection.

PREFORM: At least my theory makes a definite empirical claim. Yours has a great lacuna. You have no covering sortal. So you do not really know what you mean when you say Marie's early concept of *shmats* is the same thing as her late concept of *cats*.

EPIGEN: I accept your challenge. It won't be difficult to meet, as there seem to be several options open. Let me start with a simple suggestion, namely, that psi is a *Mental Representation*. Let 'MR', then, be the most generic sortal. Various species of MR's can be introduced later, as and when necessary. I cannot yet state explicitly the principles for counting individual MRs. But you must not demand more from me than other scientists expect from one another when they introduce theoretical sortals like 'gene' and 'quark'. Philosophers have not even succeeded in defining the precise identity conditions of *ships*! Giving precise identity conditions will require further work. But the general picture will conform to *Figure 2*, which is more biological and more parsimonious than yours.

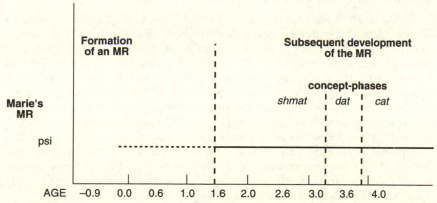

Figure 2 (*Note*. The coming-to-be of the MR is shown at around age 1.6 for the sake of the example. The actual age would need to be determined empirically.)

Let me give you an example of how a mental representation can start off undifferentiated, and can become more differentiated as time goes on. Smith, Carey and Wiser (1985) have shown that children up to seven years old have an undifferentiated concept of *weight*. They do not distinguish between an object's being *heavy* and its being *heavy for its size*. Older children, however, do succeed in distinguishing weight from density, and so their concept of *weight* is differentiated relative to the younger children's concept of *weight*. As the researchers say, 'individual concepts undergo differentiation during development' (ibid. p. 177).[17]

PREFORM: I have let you invent the name 'psi' to refer to a hypothesized continuant. But 'MR' is not a genuine covering sortal for it. An MR must have an intentional content. You can call something a representation without *mentioning* what it represents, but there has to *be* something that it represents.

Suppose for argument's sake that when psi becomes an MR it (tenselessly) represents *J*s. There will be some phase in psi's existence during which psi is a concept of *K*s, where the class of Ks is not identical with the class of Js. Yet psi is supposed to continue as an MR of *J*s throughout that phase. You are saying that psi, during that phase, both represents Ks and represents something other than Ks, which is impossible.

The example of differentiation is not apposite to your case. The undifferentiated concept and the differentiated concept have clearly distinct contents. It was only through the looseness of English that you were able to describe both of them as having the content *weight*. What you need is a covering sortal that stays true of psi *across distinct content-phases*. This requirement entails that no contentfully individuated sortal will do.

[17] Although Epigen cites this work in his support, Smith, Carey and Wiser might not endorse his ontological thesis that the older child's representation of *heaviness for size* is numerically *identical* with her own earlier representation of *heaviness*. The authors do not say that an individual concept persists across differentiation. They speak of tracing 'descent' rather than tracing identity across time; they say that the undifferentiated concept is the 'parent' of a differentiated concept, and that differentiation itself is 'the progression from a single parent to two or more descendants' (ibid. p. 179). These locutions imply that the 'parent' concept and the 'offspring' concept are numerically *distinct*, with the latter replacing the former. However, they also say 'children's concepts of weight and density do differentiate in development' (ibid. p. 178), which suggests that they take 'x is differentiated from y' to name a relation that can hold between two contemporaneous sibling concepts. Actually, it is not clear which precise proposition is expressed by the sentence 'The concept of *weight* differentiates during development'.

EPIGEN: When I say that psi is timelessly an MR, I mean that psi is an entity suitable for representing different things at different phases. If you insist on the verbal point that an MR must have content, I'll say that this MR has indeterminate content. The point is, its content is multiply determinable. It can be made determinate in one way at one time, determinate in another way at a later time. An MR is essentially an entity having certain functional properties that allow it to participate in higher cognitive processes in the distinctive way that concepts do, but it is not individuated by functional properties that fix a specific extension. It is schematic. The idea isn't unfamiliar. For example, a drawing of an animal can leave open what species the animal is. It doesn't have to represent the animal as being any particular species. But the drawing can have extra marks added which depict details (ears, whiskers, etc.) that narrow down the range of species that it could possibly represent.

For a given MR, there may be innate *constraints* upon the range of categories it can represent. Such constraints would allow the organism to adjust the MR to a specific category of things in its particular environment. Ethologists have discovered that animals are innately predisposed to learn some features of their environment more readily than they learn other features. The classes of objects to which they are especially sensitive tend to belong to biologically significant general categories, such as *food, predator, nest-site*, and so on. For example, vervet monkeys have special alarm calls for threats from the air, threats from running predators, and threats from ground-crawlers (Seyfarth, Cheney and Marler 1980). Young monkeys initially emit the signal meaning 'aerial predator' in all sorts of situations where something flies over them, including some situations where the thing is no threat. Older monkeys learn to emit the cry only when the flying object is a predatory bird of the locally prevalent kind. In one region this might be eagles, in another region hawks. Thus the representation is fine-tuned by experience so that it homes in on a specific category.

Another example is the ease with which bees learn the shapes of flowers. The bee is programmed in such a way that, whichever sort of flowers happens to be the main food source in its habitat, it forms an internal representation of that sort of flowers. This representation controls its subsequent foraging behaviour. As Gould and Marler (1987, p. 74) observe, 'In evolutionary terms innately guided learning makes sense: very often it is easy to specify in advance the general characteristics of the things an animal should be able to learn, even when the details cannot be specified.' Such developmental processes are epigenetic in the classic sense: the genes specify a range of possible trajectories, while the actual trajectory is determined by the interaction between the individual organism and its particular environment.

PREFORM: I have two objections to this story. In the first place, it does not fit the case of Marie. If her supposed MR gets more finely tuned over time, this surely means that it started off denoting a wide class, say *small furry animals*, and then it homes in on the class of *cats*. Since she had evidently linked psi to the word 'chat' by the age of 3.0, one would expect her to *overextend* 'chat' at 3.0 by applying it to any small furry animal. But in fact she *underextended* it. The concept she used was narrower in extension than a concept of *cats*; you should say that its content did not need fine-tuning, it needed broadening.

More importantly, this kind of story is in principle unable to satisfy your quest for a covering sortal that has indeterminate content. Consider the relation between the concept of *aerial predator* and the concept of *eagle*, possessed by a human subject S. Note that the former is superordinate to the latter, S has both concepts simultaneously, and they are separate. S can choose to think of Baldy the eagle in one or other guise. Your story, on the other hand, presents S's concept of *aerial predator* as the youthful version of his mature concept of *eagle*. Presumably you think that S, in his maturity, has *lost* his concept of the superordinate category! Anyway, you have not specified a content-indeterminate kind of MR; you have merely supplied an MR whose content is generic or disjunctive.

EPIGEN: Since I cannot convince you by that route, let me switch tack. You surely agree that intentional content is not a simple property. It can be split into factors. You will agree, too, that concepts can be classified into types according to various principles. The 'Different Extension' Principle (P1) is not the only one. For many explanatory purposes we classify concepts in a more finely grained way, using a 'Different Intension' Principle:

(P2) If concepts C1 and C2 have different intensions, they are distinct types.

By this test, the concepts of *salt* and *sodium chloride* are distinct, even though they are coextensive.

A third guideline that we use for some purposes is a 'Different Reference' Principle':

(P3) If concepts C1 and C2 have different referents, they are distinct types.

(P3) is compatible with a coarse-grained content taxonomy. It is sometimes acceptable to say that A's concept of London and B's concept of London are two tokens of the same type, even though A and B conceive of London somewhat differently because they have different information about the place. This is the sort of coarse concept-type that I need. For I can then say: psi is the same coarse-grained MR throughout a period in which it changes its fine-grained content.

Concepts have various semantic properties, including reference, extension, and intension. Perhaps each of these properties is itself divisible into semantic components, or into subvarieties. Philosophers have proposed a number of different theories (or notions) of *reference* and of *intension* (cf. Stich 1992). Hence it is possible for a concept to be immutable in one semantic dimension while being changeable in others.

PREFORM: What sort of coarse-content classification do you have in mind?

EPIGEN: The MRs are going to be individuated on the basis of their respective causal-historical links to their referents. Since we are talking about kind-concepts, their respective referents are categories or kinds (not individual members). When I want to refer to a category, I shall write the name of the category in capital letters.

Let us introduce the notion of an *anchoring* relation. Suppose such a relation holds at time t between a particular structure in S and an objective category K, in virtue of the fact that certain causal transactions occurred between that structure and some particular K-things prior to t. This is vague, of course; the predicate 'anchored to category K' needs to be defined more precisely. But let us suppose that this can be done. And let us further suppose that the structure in question plays an appropriate cognitive role. Then it can be said to be a representation *externally concerning* category K, where 'externally concerning' is analysed in terms of the anchoring relation. Since it is a fixed historical fact that psi became anchored to K at some time, it stays true from that time onwards that it is an MR OF K, i.e. an MR externally concerning K. The MR is individuated in terms of a naturalistic, backward-looking relational property which endows it with a 'semantic value'.

More work is required to spell out the anchoring relation. There have been several proposals in the recent philosophical literature that provide inspiration and hope. It all started with Putnam's (1975) theory of reference for natural kind terms, and with Dretske's (1981) theory of natural informational origin. Devitt and Sterelny (1987) proposed an 'aetiological' theory of reference for kind-words.

Woodfield in 1987 devised a two-tier model of concept-formation in which 'protoconcepts' (mental files) are anchored to perceptual schemas. Each schema is informationally sensitive to an observable category or property. When S attends to a particular instance of a category or property for which he has a schema, the schema is activated. When a schema is so activated, it activates the linked protoconcept. S thinks of the instance under a demonstrative mode of presentation, and the information he gleans from it is stored in the protoconcept-file dedicated to the instantiated category or property.[18]

A similarly motivated theory was proposed by Rey around the same time; details may be found in Rey (1992). Rey postulates a mental 'dthat' operator which locks the Subject on to worldly kinds and properties.

Then there are the 'teleosemantic' theories of mapping proposed by Millikan (1984), Papineau (1987) and Dretske (1988), which rely on the biological notion of proper function. Considerations of function can also be used to bolster 'aetiological' theories, as Sterelny (1990) does.

All of the above are 'locking' theories (a label coined by Rey 1992). I shall not try to adjudicate between them here. All I want to do is get across the general picture. In Marie's case, psi is an internal structure that gets anchored to the category CAT fairly early (say between one and two years of age) as a result of Marie's encounters with a small sample of cats. This link is historically fixed. From that time on, psi is an MR that externally concerns the kind CAT. In contrast, the *extension* of psi (at a given time) is the set of objects to which Marie would be disposed to apply psi at that time. Her disposition is trainable, hence the extension varies as time goes on. If we distinguish concept-types in accordance with the 'Different Extension' Principle, psi instantiates distinct concepts at different times. And of course, if we distinguish concepts according to the 'Different Intension' Principle, psi's life-history is divided into even finer concept-phases. Yet throughout these phases psi remains continuously an MR OF CAT (see *Figure 3*).

PREFORM: Why do you say that psi at age 3.0 was anchored in the category CAT, as opposed to being anchored in the category SHMAT? The causal transactions she had with a few local cats were also, equally, transactions with local shmats. In fact, there are indefinitely many ways of generalizing from that small set of ani-

---

[18] The 'Schemas and Protoconcepts' theory was presented at various seminars and conferences between 1987 and 1989; for contractual reasons the only published version (Woodfield 1992) is in French. Woodfield (1987) set out some of the motivations for the theory; later work expressed scepticism about the notion of 'mental file' (see Woodfield 1991).

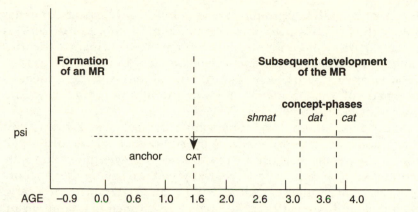

Figure 3 (*Note.* Dating the moment of anchoring at around 1.6 is, again, merely an illustrative hypothesis).

mals to categories that they all belonged to. You seem to be giving priority to one category over the others. Is it because cats form a natural kind, whereas shmats do not? If that's your reason, it's a bad one. You ought not to favour natural kind concepts in that way; most concepts are not natural kind concepts. You have no reason to assume that psi is destined to be one.

Suppose Marie lived in a culture where shmats were thought to constitute a category, lexically marked by 'chat'. Would you still say that psi was anchored in CAT? No. You would try to make out that it was anchored in SHMAT. You would want to fix things so that the anchoring category coincided with the category that would be mentally represented by the concept when it was 'mature'. The anchor is indeed 'fixed'—fixed by you, with the benefit of hindsight!

EPIGEN: Not at all. I am supposing that we can identify psi's anchoring category at the toddler stage, independently of our guess about where psi will end up. There is no preestablished harmony, no guarantee that any concept possessed by a child will actually reach maturity. What is true, however, is that my *criterion of maturity* for any given MR is met when its extension has stabilized on the class of objects that belong to the category to which it was originally anchored.

I admit that I have not explained precisely what it is for an MR to be locked on to a determinate general category or property in the world. As I said, there are several alternative proposals currently being explored. The business proves to be rather complicated; each proposal seems to run up against the same sorts of problems. For informational semantics there is the problem of misinformation, and the problem of characterizing the process of locking on during the 'learning-period'. These are aspects of what Fodor calls 'the disjunction problem' (Fodor 1988). For direct reference theories, there is the *qua* problem. Teleosemantic theories also have problems of content-indeterminacy. For Rey there is the problem of fortuitous lockings. But the authors of these theories are aware of the problems and are intent upon solving them. Progress is being made!

PREFORM: I doubt that. The whole project seems beset with insuperable internal problems. Nevertheless, I shan't press you now on the details, because I want to keep our eyes glued on to the central *developmental* issue. Essentially you are saying that anchoring gives psi enough semantics to be an MR, and that coarse semantic stability enables psi to change its extension and intension while remaining numerically the same MR. It is interesting that you, in your move to fix psi semantically, are getting close to my preformationist view. I say that the mental content of a given concept is immutable from birth; you now say that the coarse content of psi is immutable from the time at which psi becomes anchored. We now agree that a concept cannot be identified except as having *some sort* of content which never changes.

But does this last-ditch strategy buy you what you really want? Surely your original problem, of finding a content-neutral covering-sortal, pops up again at an earlier age! You want to trace the development of psi across time. You accept that you need a covering sortal that spans any two moments of psi's existence. You say that psi acquires an anchor at some time before Marie is 3.0, and that this is the time when psi becomes an MR. What sort of thing is psi *before that time*? Not a representation at all. Thus the diachronic identity problem now gets concentrated upon that crucial phase of development spanning the period from psi's coming to be up to the time when psi's anchor is fixed. This is the process of psi's *becoming an MR*. If this is a genuine developmental process, there has to be a principle for individuating the thing that undergoes this transformation.

EPIGEN: The very early phase to which you refer is indeed crucial. What happens in that phase is the *formation* of an MR. As embryologists know, the forming of a T-thing can be either the coming into existence of an individual, or a pre-existing individual becoming a T-thing. So one hypothesis is that *psi* comes into existence during that phase. On this view, psi is an MR anchored in CATS from the first moment of its existence. But I want to resist that hypothesis, because it implies content-preformationism. I want to stick to the view that psi acquires representational status during its lifetime.

It looks as though I am forced to find a covering sortal that does not characterize psi as essentially a contentful thing. No kind of content, however primitive, can be individuative of psi. So, instead of calling psi a Mental Representation, I shall call it a Cognitive Structure. Criteria of identity for CS's will be provided later, when I have done more work. The appropriate level of classification, the vocabulary from which I shall draw, will not be mentalistic, and it will not be neurophysiological, but it will be at a level intermediate between these. Perhaps psi is essentially and timelessly an individual of a purely syntactic kind. Or maybe it is a computational structure, such as a frame or a Q-morphism, or something.

PREFORM: Maybe that is your best bet. Your postulated continuant had better not be identified with any particular *anatomical* structure, since a computational entity might be realized in different neural circuits at different times. It is not likely that spatiotemporal continuity will figure as a criterion for the identity of an individual CS. But remember, 'Cognitive Structure' is just a promissory note, a dummy sortal. You have no idea how to trace a particular Cognitive Structure across time. You pretend that there is some principle. But there is not.

IV. Escape From The Debate

In the dialectic between Epigen and Preform, neither side won. Epigen's efforts to find a genuine covering sortal met with no success. Preform's position was no more than a debating stance, for his claim that all concepts are innate is surely false. It is time to consider the possibility that they are both making a mistake. Since they share several assumptions in virtue of their commitment to the IRTC, perhaps one or more of those common assumptions is false.

I want to suggest that the most fundamental error which both parties make is to believe that a personal concept is a particular. Epigen thought, and Preform went along with the thought, that they were referring to a determinate internal particular, which they designated with the name 'psi'. The debate was about what *kind* of particular psi might substantially be. But do we need to suppose that a personal concept is an internal particular in order to make sense of the real issues in developmental psychology? The subject-matter of developmental psychology is not so concrete as the subject-matter of embryology; perhaps the notions of growth and development need to be construed in a more abstract way.

Consider two embryologists examining a foetus whose growth they have both traced from the zygote. Suppose they disagree about the time at which a particular limb, which they decide to call 'lambda', was first formed. More specifically, they disagree about the appropriate criteria for deciding when something is truly a limb (and not merely a limb-bud). The ordinary word 'limb' is not precise enough for their purposes; consulting a dictionary will not help them to resolve their dispute. And Nature provides no sharp demarcating moment in the growth of a limb-bud. It is a taxonomic dispute rather than a merely semantic dispute, and it may have important theoretical implications for them. One thing they do agree on, however, is that there is a particular object, lambda, which they are both referring to and disputing about.

Now imagine two developmentalists engaged in a superficially similar argument about the moment when a child first attained a certain concept, say the concept of *liquid*. A great deal of the literature in developmental psychology is devoted to answering questions of this type. For example, Spelke's work on very young infants shows that babies have expectations about the cohesion and boundedness, the substantiality and the persistence of solid objects, even before they have had time to learn about objects through manipulation. Spelke (1988) concluded that infants around 4 months old possess a concept which approximates to the concept of *object*. This conflicts with Piaget's claim that children attain the *object*-concept at around 2 years of age. Spelke's experimental evidence was not available to Piaget; indeed the habituation-dishabituation technique that she used was unknown or unfeasible in his day. It is conceivable that if Piaget had been aware of Spelke's data, he would have agreed with her conclusion. But the choice between two hypotheses about the age of attainment is not always resolvable by obtaining more data. Psychologists often disagree about how to *interpret* the behavioural data. The debate about when children attain the *object* concept has been dogged by fundamental disagreements of this sort.

So imagine that our two psychologists share precisely the same information about the behaviour of the two year old child whom they are studying. Yet one maintains that such behaviour is proof that the child has attained the concept of *liquid*, while the other regards that same behaviour as proof that she is still in the process of forming it.

Is this parallel to the dispute between the two embryologists? It might seem so at first sight. It might seem that the two psychologists disagree, with respect to a particular cognitive structure inside the two year old, about whether that structure counts as a concept of *liquid*. If you take the embryological analogy seriously, you are tempted to think that there was a *thing* that the psychologists were both referring to, just as the embryologists were co-referring to an observed cell-cluster. But this is not so. There is no independently identifiable referent such that psychologists disagree about how to classify it. The only question at issue between them is: what are the conditions that children must meet in order for them to be said to conceptualize liquids as *liquids*? This is a question about the conditions for being conceptually competent in a certain way. It does not refer to, or quantify over, concept-particulars.

Peacocke (1989) asserts a principle: there can be no more to a theory of a given concept other than a theory of what it is for a person to possess that concept. Peacocke is talking about Fregean concepts, not personal concepts, but we can adapt his principle to our present discussion. For it has the corollary, I take it, that certain kinds of numerical identity questions do not arise. Instead of trying to trace a particular concept across time, we need only follow the career of a person and chart his or her transition from being a non-possessor to being a possessor. The development is adequately described in terms of the person's changing abilities and changing relationships.

It is possible to cite many passages from the literature which appear to assume that S's concept of such-and-such is a persisting particular inside S's head. Yet I suggest that the cognitive developmental issues that really interest psychologists are expressible in language that is not ontologically committed to such things. I put this forward as a suggestion; I do not claim to have proved it. A proper defense would require a thorough survey of the many problems which developmentalists try to address. But if my suggestion is correct, if it is indeed a mistake to reify personal concepts, this would account for the air of unreality which surrounds the debate between Epigen and Preform.

It is important to stress that the suggestion in no way stems from a hostility to internal representations in *general*. On the contrary, I maintain that any being who has concepts *must* have internal representations. Also, in order for a person to have a concept of Ks, it is necessary that there be some persisting inner structures that are specific markers of, *proof* of, possession of that concept. The point is simply that none of these structures *is* S's concept of Ks.

There is no space for me to expound my positive views here. I shall conclude, then, by urging that the process of conceptual development in children be reconceptualised. It is not a biological process like the growth of organs. Biologism in psychology breeds an inappropriate concretism, and nowhere is this inappropriateness more dramatically felt than in the domain of developmental phenomena.

References

Brennan, A. 1988. *Conditions of Identity*. Oxford: Clarendon Press.

Carey, S. 1985. *Conceptual Change in Childhood*. Cambridge, MA: MIT Press.

Carey, S. 1988. 'Conceptual differences between children and adults', *Mind and Language*, **3**, 3, 167–181.

Carterette, E.C. and Friedman, M. P. 1973. (eds.) *Handbook of Perception. Vol III: Biology of Perceptual Systems*. New York and London: Academic Press.

Devitt, M. and Sterelny, K. 1987. *Language and Reality*. Oxford: Blackwell.

Dretske, F. 1981. *Knowledge and the Flow of Information*. Oxford: Blackwell.

Dretske, F. 1988. *Explaining Behavior: Reasons in a World of Causes*. Cambridge, MA: MIT Press.

Fodor, J. A. 1980. 'Fixation of belief and concept acquisition' (and ensuing discussion), in M. Piattelli-Palmarini (1980), pp. 143–158.

Fodor, J. A. 1981. 'The present status of the innateness controversy', in *Representations* ch. 10, pp. 257–316. Brighton: Harvester Press.

Fodor, J. 1988. *Psychosemantics*. Cambridge, MA: MIT Press.

Gould, J. L. & Marler, P. 1987. 'Learning by instinct', *Scientific American*, **256**, 74–85

Keil, F. C. 1989. *Concepts, Kinds and Cognitive Development*. Cambridge MA: MIT Press.

Macnamara, J. 1986. *A Border Dispute: The Place of Logic in Psychology*. Cambridge, MA: MIT Press.

McShane, J. 1991. *Cognitive Development: An Information Processing Approach*. Oxford: Blackwell.

Millikan, R. 1984. *Language, Thought, and Other Biological Categories*. Cambridge, MA: MIT Press.

Papineau, D. 1987. *Reality and Representation*. Oxford: Blackwell.

Peacocke, C. 1989. *Transcendental Arguments in the Theory of Content*. Oxford: Oxford University Press.

Piaget, J. 1973. *Autobiography,* in R. I. Evans (ed.) *Jean Piaget, the Man and his Ideas*. New York: Dutton.

Piattelli-Palmarini, M. 1980 (ed.) *Language and Learning*. London and Henley: Routledge and Kegan Paul.

Putnam, H. 1975. 'The meaning of "meaning"', in *Mind, Language, and Reality (Philosophical Papers vol. II)*. Cambridge: Cambridge University Press.

Rey, G. 1992. 'Semantic externalism and conceptual competence', *Proceedings of the Aristotelian Society,* **XCII**, 3, 315–333.

Seyfarth, R., Cheney, D. L. and Marler, P. 1980. 'Monkey responses to three different alarm calls: Evidence of predator classification and semantic communication', *Science,* **210**, 801–803.

Smith, C., Carey, S. and Wiser, M. 1985. 'On differentiation: A case study of the development of the concepts of size, weight, and density', *Cognition,* **21**, 177–237.

Sober, E. 1984. *The Nature of Selection*. Cambridge, MA: MIT Press.

Spelke, E. 1988. 'The origins of physical knowledge', in L. Weiskrantz (ed.) *Thought Without Language*. Oxford: Clarendon Press.

Sterelny, K. 1990. *The Representational Theory of Mind* Oxford: Blackwell.

Stich, S. P. 1992. 'What is a theory of mental representation?', *Mind, 101*, 402, 243–261.

Trevarthen, C. B.1973. 'Behavioral embryology', in Carterette and Friedman (1973), chapter 5, pp. 89–117.

Waddington, C. 1966. *Principles of Development and Differentiation*. London: Collier-MacMillan.

Wiggins, D. 1980. *Sameness and Substance*. Oxford: Blackwell.

Woodfield, A. 1976. *Teleology*. Cambridge: Cambridge University Press.

Woodfield, A. 1987. 'On the very idea of acquiring a concept', in J. Russell (ed.) *Philosophical Perspectives on Developmental Psychology*, pp.17–30. Oxford: Blackwell.

Woodfield, A. 1991. 'Conceptions', in *Mind and Content, Mind,* **C**, 4, 547–572.

Woodfield, A. 1992. 'Un modèle à deux étapes de la formation des concepts', in Daniel Andler (ed.) *Introduction aux sciences cognitives*, pp. 273–290. Paris: Gallimard.

Woodger, J. H. 1929. *Biological Principles*. London: Kegan Paul, Trench, Trubner.

The Mind as a Control System*

AARON SLOMAN

1. Introduction

This is not a scholarly research paper, but a 'position paper' outlining an approach to the study of mind which has been gradually evolving (at least in my mind) since about 1969 when I first become acquainted with work in Artificial Intelligence through Max Clowes. I shall try to show why it is more fruitful to construe the mind as a control system than as a computational system (although computation can play a role in control mechanisms).

During the 1970s and most of the 1980s I was convinced that the best way to think of the human mind was as a computational system, a view that I elaborated in my book *The Computer Revolution in Philosophy* published in 1978. (Though I did point out that there were many aspects of human intelligence whose explanation and simulation were still a very long way off.)

At that time I thought I knew exactly what I meant by 'computational' but during the late 1980s, while trying to write a second book (still unfinished), I gradually became aware that I was confused between two concepts. On the one hand there is a very precisely definable technical concept of computation, such as is studied in mathematical computer science (which is essentially concerned with *syntactic* relations between sequences of structures, e.g. formally definable states of a machine or sets of symbols), and on the other hand there is a more intuitive, less well-defined concept such as people use when they ask what computation a part of the brain performs, or when they think of a computer as essentially a machine that *does* things under the *control* of one or more programs. The second concept is used when we talk about analog computers, for these involve continuous variation of voltages, currents, and the like, and so there are no sequences of states.

Attempting to resolve the confusion revealed that there were not merely two but several different notions of computation that might be referred to in claiming that the mind is a computational system. Many of the arguments for and against the so-called 'Strong AI

* I am grateful for comments and criticisms of earlier versions of this paper and related papers, made by colleagues and students in the Cognitive Science Research Centre, the University of Birmingham.

Thesis' muddle up these different concepts and are therefore at cross purposes, arguing for not inconsistent positions, despite the passion in the conflicts, as I've tried to show in (Sloman 1992), which demonstrates that there are at least eight different interpretations of the thesis, some obviously true, some obviously false, and some still open to investigation.

Eventually I realized that the non-technical concept of computation was too general, too ill-defined, and too unconstrained to have explanatory power: whereas the essentially syntactic technical concept was too narrow: there was no convincing reason to believe that being a certain sort of computation in that sense was either necessary or sufficient for the replication of human-like mentality, no matter which computation it was.

Being entirely computational in the technical sense could not be necessary for mentality because the technical notion requires all processes to be discrete whereas there is no good reason why continuous mechanisms and processes should not play a significant part in the way a mind works, along with discrete processes.

Being a computation in the technical sense could not be sufficient for production of mental states either. On the contrary, a static sequence of formulae written on sheets of paper could satisfy the narrow *technical* definition of 'computation' whereas a mind is essentially something that involves processes that interact causally with one another.

To see that causation is not part of the technical concept of computation, consider that the limit theorems showing that certain sorts of computations cannot exist merely show that certain sequences of formulae, or sequences of ordered structures (machine states) cannot exist, e.g. sequences of Turing machine states that generate non-computable decimal numbers. The famous proofs produced by Gödel, Turing, Tarski and others do not need to make assumptions about causal powers of machines in order to derive non-computability results. Similarly complexity results concerning the number of steps required for certain computations, or the number of co-existing memory locations do not need to make any assumptions about causation. Neither would adding any assumptions about computation as involving causation make any difference to those results. Even the definition of a Turing machine requires only that it has a sequence of states that conform to the machine's transition table: there is no requirement that this conformity be *caused* or *controlled* by anything, not even any mechanism implementing the transition table. All the mathematical proofs about properties and limitations of Turing machines and other computers depend only on the formal or syntactic relations between sequences of states. There is not even a requirement that the states occur in a temporal sequence. The proofs would apply equally to static, coexisting, sequences of marks on paper that were isomorphic to the succession of states in time. The proofs can even apply to sequences of states encoded as Gödel numbers that exist neither in space nor in time, but are purely abstract. This argument is elaborated in Sloman (1992), as part of a demonstration that there is an interpretation of the Strong AI thesis in which it is trivially false and not worth arguing about. This version of the thesis, I suspect, is the one that Searle thinks he has refuted (Searle 1980), though I don't think any researchers in AI actually believe it. There are other, more interesting versions that are left untouched by the 'Chinese Room' argument.

Unfortunately, the broader, more intuitive concept of computation seems to be incapable of being defined with sufficient precision to form the basis for an interesting, non-circular, conjecture about the nature of mind. For example, if it turns out that in this intuitive sense *everything* is a computer (as I once conjectured, perhaps foolishly, (Sloman 1978)), then saying that a mind is a computer says nothing about what distinguishes minds (or the brains that implement them) from other behaving systems, such as clouds or falling rocks.

I conclude that, although concepts and techniques from computer science have played a powerful catalytic role in expanding our ideas about mental mechanisms, it is a mistake to try to link the notion of mentality too closely to the notion of computation. In fact, doing so generates apparently endless and largely fruitless debates between people talking at cross purposes without realizing it.

Instead, all that is needed for a scientific study of the mind is the assumption that there is a class of *mechanisms* that can be shown to be capable of producing all the known phenomena. There is no need for researchers in AI, cognitive science or philosophy to make restrictive assumptions about such mechanisms, such as that they must be purely computational, especially when that claim is highly ambiguous. Rather we should try to characterize suitable classes of mechanisms at the highest level of generality and then expand with as much detail as is needed for our purposes, making no prior commitments that are not entailed by the requirements for the particular mechanisms proposed. We may then discover that different sorts of mechanisms are capable of producing different sorts of minds, and that could be a significant contribution to an area of biology that until now appears not to have produced any hard theories: the evolution of mind and behaviour.

2. How can we make progress?

When trying to find a general starting point for a theory about the nature of minds there are many options. Some philosophers start from the notion of 'rationality', or from a small number of familiar aspects of human mentality, such as beliefs and desires, or something common to several of them, often referred to as 'intentionality.' I suggest that it would be more fruitful to step back to the very general notion of a mechanism that interacts with a changing environment, including parts of itself, in a way that is determined by (a) the changeable internal state of the mechanism, (b) the state of the environment and (c) the history of previous interactions (through which the internal state gets changed). This is a deeply *causal* concept, the concept of a *control system*. So I am proposing that we revive some old ideas and elaborate on the not particularly novel thesis that the mind is essentially a control system. But this is still too general, for the notion of such a control system covers many physical objects (both naturally occurring or manufactured) that clearly lack minds. By adding extra constraints to this general concept we may be able to home in on a set of interesting special cases, more or less like human beings or other animals.

The purposes for which mental phenomena are studied and explained will vary from one discipline to another. In the case of AI, the ultimate requirement is to produce working models with human-like mental properties, whether in order to provide detailed scientific explanations or in order to solve practical problems. For psychologists the goal may be to model very specific details of human performance, including details that differ from one individual to another, or from one experimental situation to another. For engineering applications of AI, the goal will be to produce working systems that perform very specific classes of tasks in well-specified environments. In the case of philosophy it will normally suffice to explore the *general* nature of the mechanisms underlying mental phenomena down to a level that makes clear how those mechanisms are capable of accounting for the peculiar features of machines that can think, feel, take decisions, and so on.

That is the goal of this paper, though in other contexts it would be preferable to expand to a lower level of detail and even show how to produce a working system, in a manner that would satisfy the needs of both applied AI and detailed psychological modelling.

Since there are many kinds of control systems, I shall have to say what's special about a mind. I shall also try to indicate where computation fits into this framework. I'll start by summarizing some alternative approaches with which this approach can be contrasted.

3. Philosophical approaches to mind

Philosophers generally try to study the mind by using conceptual and logical approaches, with subtasks such as the following:

- Analyse ordinary concepts to define notions like 'mind', 'consciousness', 'pleasure', 'pain', etc.
- Attempt to produce arguments ('transcendental deductions' Kant called them) showing that certain things are absolutely necessary for some aspect of mind or other.
- Produce metaphysical theories about what kinds of things need to exist in order to make minds possible (e.g. different kinds of stuff, special kinds of causal relationships, etc.)

Further common philosophical questions include whether all mental phenomena can be reduced to some subset (e.g. whether all mental states can be defined in terms of collections of beliefs and desires), whether certain descriptions of mental phenomena are names of 'natural kinds', which phenomena can be assessed as rational or irrational, and whether it is possible to know the contents of another person's mind.

It is very hard to discuss or evaluate such analyses and theories, e.g. because

- Ordinary concepts are full of imprecision and indeterminacy limiting their technical usefulness. So questions posed in terms of them may lack determinate answers.
- The theories usually have a level of generality and imprecision that makes it very hard to assess their implications or evaluate them. Acceptance or rejection appears often to be a matter of personal taste or prejudice, or philosophical fashion.
- It is hard to distinguish substantive questions with true or false answers from questions that are to be answered by taking more or less arbitrary terminological decisions (e.g. where are the boundaries between emotions, moods, attitudes, or between animals that are and animals that are not conscious?)
- Very often the philosophical issues are posed in terms of a small subset of the known phenomena of mind (e.g. conscious thought

73

processes expressible in words) whereas any theory of what minds are and how they work should encompass far more richness, including indescribably rich experiences (like watching a waterfall), and phenomena exhibited only in young children, people with brain damage, and in some cases other animals.

- The variety found in animals of various sorts, human infants, brain damaged people, etc. suggests that there are few or no absolutely necessary conditions for the existence of mental capabilities, only a collection of different designs with different properties.

- Philosophers often make false assumptions about what sorts of mechanisms can or cannot exist because they have not been trained as software engineers and therefore know only about limited classes of mechanisms and have only very crude conceptions of possible computational mechanisms. In particular, they tend to be ignorant of the way in which the concept of a 'virtual machine' has extended our ideas. (A virtual machine is created in a physical machine by programs such as 'interpreters' that make it possible to specify higher level machines that have totally different properties from the physical machine. In a machine running text-processing software such as I am now using, there are letters, numerals, words, sentences, paragraphs, diagrams, chapters, etc., and there are mechanisms for operating on these things, e.g. by inserting, deleting, or re-ordering these objects. However these textual entities are not physical entities and do not exist in the physical computer, which remains the same machine when the word-processing software is replaced by some other software, e.g. a circuit design package.)

These are among the features of philosophical discussion that often provoke exasperated impatience among non-philosophers, e.g. scientists interested in the study of mind who encounter phenomena that are ignored by philosophers, including other animals, people with brain damage and sophisticated machines.

The real determinants of the mind are not conceptual requirements such as rationality, but biological and engineering design requirements, concerned with issues like speed, flexibility, appropriateness to the environment, coping with limited resources, information retention capabilities, etc. We'll get further if we concentrate more on how it is possible for a machine to match its internal and external processes to the fine structure of a fast-moving environment, and less on what it is to be rational or conscious. Properties such as rationality and intentionality will then emerge if we get our designs right. 'Consciousness' will probably turn out to be a concept that's too ill-defined to be of any use: it will instead be replaced by a collection of systematically generated concepts derived from theoretical analysis of what different control systems can do.

4. Philosophers as designers

For the reasons given above, my preferred approach to many philosophical questions is to treat them from the standpoint of an engineer trying to design something more or less like a human being, but without assuming that there's going to be only *one* possible design, or that there are any absolutely necessary conditions to be satisfied, or even that the notion of what is to be designed is precisely specified in advance. I call this the 'design-based' approach (defined more fully in Sloman (1993)).

This is closely related to what Dennett described as the 'design stance' (Dennett 1978). It requires us to specify our theories from the standpoint of how things work: how perception works, how motives are generated, how decisions are taken, how learning occurs, and so on. Moreover, it requires us to specify these designs with sufficient clarity and precision that a future engineer might be able to expand them into a working instantiation. Since this is very difficult to do, we may, for a while, only be able to *approximate* the task, or achieve it only for *fragments* of mental processes, which is what has happened in AI so far.

But the design stance does not require unique solutions to design problems. We must keep an open mind as to whether there are alternative designs with interestingly varied properties: abandoning Kant's idea of a 'transcendental deduction' proving that certain features are necessary. Instead we can explore the structure of 'design space' to find out what sorts of behaving systems are possible, and how they differ.

Adopting this stance teaches us that our ordinary concepts are inadequate to cope with the full variety of kinds of systems and kinds of capabilities, states, or behaviour that can emerge from exploratory studies of alternative designs in various kinds of environments, just as they are inadequate for categorizing the full variety of forms of mind found in biological organisms, including microbes, insects, rodents, chimps and human beings. If we don't yet know what mechanisms there may be, nor what processes they can produce, we can't expect our language to be able to describe and accurately distinguish all the interestingly different cases that can occur, any more than ordinary concepts can provide a basis for saying when a foetus becomes a human being or when someone with severe brain damage is no longer a human being. Our concepts did not evolve to be capable of dealing with such cases.

We should assess theories in terms of their ability to support designs that actually work, as opposed to merely satisfying rationality requirements, fitting introspection, or 'sounding convincing' to willing believers.

In true philosophical spirit we can let our designs, and our theorizing, range over the full space of possibilities instead of being constrained to consider only designs for systems that already exist: this exploration of possible alternatives is essential for clarifying our concepts and deepening our understanding of existing systems.

This is very close to the approach of AI, especially broad-minded versions of AI that make no assumptions regarding mechanisms to be used. Both computational and non-computational mechanisms may be relevant, though it's not obvious that there's a sharp distinction.

5. Key ideas, and some implications

I'll now try to list some of the key ideas driving the design-based study of mind.

- A mind is a well-designed, sophisticated, self-modifying control system, with functional requirements such as speed, flexibility, adaptability, generality, precision and autonomous generation of goals. It is able to operate in a richly structured, only partly accessible, fast-changing environment in which some active entities are also minds.
- This idea, that a mind is a control system meeting complex, detailed and stringent engineering requirements, when developed in full detail, has profound implications for several theoretical and scientific disciplines concerned with the study of aspects of the human mind, such as philosophy, psychology and linguistics: it suggests the form that explanatory theories have to take, and it has implications regarding evaluation of theories. For instance, it is not enough for a theory to be consistent with observed behaviour: Additional possible criteria can be explored such as (a) that the design should use 'low level' mechanisms like those found in brains, or (b) that the design should be capable of having been produced by an evolutionary process, or (c) that it must be a *good* design.
- By exploring different criteria of goodness for designs we can replace the impoverished philosophical criteria for agency, such

as rationality or consciousness with a host of different sorts of requirements, including speed and flexibility, and explore their consequences.

- All this has practical implications, for education, counselling, and the design of usable interactive systems: for it is only when you understand how something works that you can understand ways in which it can go wrong, or design good strategies for dealing with it.

- The view that a mind is a control system is not provable or refutable: it defines an approach to the study of mind. In particular, it is not possible to argue against those who believe minds include a 'magical' element inaccessible except through introspection and inexplicable by scientific (mechanistic) theories of mind: that sort of belief is not rationally discussable. I shall simply ignore it here, though I think it can sometimes be overcome by a long sequence of personal philosophical 'tutorials', partly analogous to therapy.

- An *intelligent* control system will differ in important ways from the kinds of control systems hitherto studied by mathematicians and engineers. For instance, much of the control is concerned with how information is processed, rather than with how physical factors, such as force or speed, are varied. This point is developed below.

- By surveying types of control systems, their properties, the kinds of states they can have, we may expect to generate a 'rational reconstruction' of concepts currently used for describing mental states and processes, analogous to the way the periodic table of chemical elements led to a rational reconstruction of pre-scientific concepts of kinds of stuff. In both cases, primitive but usable collections of pre-theoretic concepts evolve gradually into more systematic families of concepts corresponding to configurations of states and processes compatible with a deep theory.

- In particular, the idea of a mind as control system leads to a new analysis of the concept of 'representation': a representation is part of a control state: and different kinds of representations play different roles in control mechanisms. (There are many different kinds of representations, useful for different purposes, each with its own syntax, semantics, and manipulation mechanisms.)

- Some AI work has concentrated excessively on representations (formalisms) and algorithms required for particular tasks, such as planning, reasoning, visual perception or language understanding. We also need to consider global *architectures* combining several different functions and we need to explore varieties of mechanisms within which such architectures can be implemented. This means considering not only what information is used, how it is represented and how it is transformed, but also what the important functional components of the system are, and what their causal powers and functional roles are in the system. Much of the functionality can be circular: the function of A is partly to modify the behaviour of B, and the function of B is partly to modify the behaviour of A. (Beliefs and desires are related in this circular fashion, which is why purely behavioural analyses of mental states fail.)

- From the standpoint outlined here, some debates about the relative merits of connectionist mechanisms and symbol-processing mechanisms appear trivial, for they are concerned with 'low level' details, whereas it is more important to understand the global architectures capable of supporting mind-like properties. I suspect that we shall find that, as in many control systems, architecture dominates mechanism: that is, changing the low level implementation details will make only a marginal difference to the capabilities of the system at least in normal circumstances.

- In an intelligent control system most of the important processes are likely to be found in abstract or 'virtual' machines, whose main features are not physical properties and physical behaviour, though they are *implemented* in terms of lower level physical machines. The virtual machines manipulate complex information structures (such as networks of symbols) rather than physical objects and their physical properties. For example, a word-processor manipulates words, paragraphs, etc., though these cannot be found in the underlying physical machine. Similarly, although they interact causally, the components of a virtual machine do not interact via physical causes, such as forces, voltages, pressures, magnetic fields, even though they are implemented in terms of machines that do.

This last point, I believe, is the most important contribution of computer science to the philosophical study of mind, rather than the concept of a program or algorithm that generates behaviour, though much discussion of the relevance of computation has focused on the latter.

6. What distinguishes mind-like control systems?

Suppose we think of a mind as: an incredibly complex, self-monitoring, self-modifying control system, implemented at least in part as a collection of interacting virtual machines. This raises the following question, already hinted at: How is it like and how is it unlike other control systems? For instance, there is a large body of mathematics concerning control systems, usually represented as a set of measurable quantities and a set of differential equations stating how those quantities change over time. Does that help us understand how minds work? I believe the answer turns out to be: 'not much'! This is for the following reasons:

- The most important changes and processes in a mind don't map onto numeric variation: many of the architectural changes and the processes that occur within components of the architecture are *structural*, not quantitative. For example, they may involve the creation and modification of structures like trees and networks, for instance parse-trees representing perceptual structures. By contrast the typical components of an unintelligent control mechanism will be concerned with varying some measurable quantity, and even if there are many quantities sensed or modified, and many links between them, the variety of causal roles is limited to what can be expressed by sets of partial differential equations linking changing numerical measures. This does not allow for processes like creation of a parse-tree when a sentence is analysed or creation of a structural description when a retinal image is interpreted. (This point is rather subtle: I am not denying that mechanisms of the required type can be virtual machines that are *implemented* in mechanisms of the wrong type: a pattern that pervades computer science and software engineering.)
- The architecture of a human mind is so rich: there's enormous functional differentiation within each individual. Not only are there many different components to a working human-like mind, they have very different functional roles, including analysing and interpreting sensory input, generating new motives, creating and executing plans, creating representations of possible futures, storing information for future use, forming new generalizations, and many more. These differences of function are not easily captured by standard mathematical formalisms for representing changing systems.
- The architecture of an intelligent, human-like system is not static, it develops over time. A child gradually develops new combinations of capabilities concerned with cognitive skills, and also motivational and emotional control. A fixed set of differential equations can't model a changing architecture. Even if the architecture at a particular time could be expressed by such a set of equations, something more would be needed to represent the change from one set of equations to another, and that's not something differential equations can do (though it can be done by symbol manipulating programs). This point is not unique to mind-like control sys-

tems: it is commonplace in biological systems, where seeds change into trees, caterpillars change into moths and every embryo has a rapidly changing structure. The architectural changes in a human mind are more subtle and far harder to detect than structural changes in organisms, especially if they are changes in virtual machine structures without any simple physical correlates.

All of this implies that:

- Causal influences are not all expressible as transmission of measurable quantities like force, current, etc. Some involve transmission of structured 'messages' and instructions between sub-components. Some processes build new structures. Some of the causal interactions occur in the virtual machines that are supervenient on physical machines. (I am aware that some philosophers believe that supervenient processes cannot interact causally. It would take too long to refute that here: what happens in software systems is a concrete refutation.)
- New kinds of mathematics are needed to cope with this, although there has been some progress already, for example in the mathematical study of formal languages, proof systems, parsing mechanisms, and transformations of datastructures.
- Most of the control systems previously studied by mathematicians and engineers do not involve operations in virtual machines: they are physical machines with physical processes that are controlled by other physical processes. Thus the basic processes are expressible as physical laws relating physical quantities. In a mind the processes occur in a variety of virtual machines whose laws differ greatly. The processes involved in creating a 3-D interpretation from a 2-D image, and the processes involved in deriving a new plan of action from a set of beliefs and goals are very different from each other and from the way changes in temperature can produce changes in pressure or volume.

The currently fashionable ideas from dynamical systems theory are unlikely to prove rich enough to fill the need. I shall try to explain why in the next section.

7. The need for new concepts

We need new thinking tools to help us grasp all this complexity. We lack good 'global ideas' to help us think about the architecture of the whole mind: how the bits studied by AI fit together. A key idea is that a control system has independently variable causally interacting sub-states. By looking at ways in which complex systems can be analysed into components with their own changing states with different characteristics, we can begin to describe global architectures. For this purpose we should not think of a behaving system as having a single 'atomic' total state that changes over time, as is common in physics and engineering. Rather we need the notion of a 'molecular' state, which is made of several different states that can change separately.

- *atomic state*: The whole system state is thought of as indivisible, and the system moves from one state to another through a 'state space' sometimes referred to as a 'phase space'. The total system has a single 'trajectory' in state space. There may be 'attractors', that is regions of state space which, once reached, cannot be left.

The idea of a complete system as having an atomic state with a 'trajectory' in phase space is an old idea in physics, but it may not be the most useful way to think about a system that is made of many interacting subsystems. For example a typical modern computer can be thought of as having a state represented by a vector giving the bit-values of all the locations in its memory and in its registers, and all processes in the computer can be thought of in terms of the trajectory of that state-vector in the machine's state space. However, in practice this has not proved a useful way for software engineers to think about the behaviour of the computer. Rather it is generally more useful to think of various persisting sub-components (strings, arrays, trees, networks, databases, stored programs) as having their own changing states which interact with one another.

So it is often more useful to consider separate subsystems as having their own states, especially when the architecture changes, so that the set of subsystems, and substates, is not static but new ones can be created and old ones removed. This leads to the following notion:

- *molecular state with sub-states*: The instantaneous state of a complete system sometimes includes many coexisting, independently variable, interacting, states of different kinds, which change in different ways, under external or internal influences. These may be states of subsystems with very different functional roles. The number of relevant interacting substates may change over time, as a result of their interactions.

A physicist or engineer who represents a complex system by a vector of measurements representing a point in a high dimensional 'phase space' and treats all change as motion of the point is using the *atomic* notion of a state. By contrast, if the system is thought of as having many different components and the processes of change in those components are studied separately, the concept of state is then *molec-*

ular. Of course, if the atomic state is represented by a vector there are independently variable components: the components of the vector. But in a molecular state the number of components and their connections can vary over time, and some of the components will themselves have complex molecular states; whereas for atomic states the number of dimensions of a phase space is fixed, and the components of the vectors are numerical values rather than complex structures. Thus the molecular conception of state allows the state of a system to be hierarchically structured, with changing structures at several levels in the hierarchy.

Within the molecular approach we can identify a variety of functional sub-divisions between sub-states and sub-mechanisms, and investigate different kinds of functional and causal interactions. For example, we can describe part of the system as a long term information store, another part as a short-term buffer for incoming information, another as concerned with interpreting sensory input, another as drawing implications from previously acquired information, another as storing goals waiting to be processed, and so on. The notion of a global atomic state with a single trajectory is particularly unhelpful where the various components of the system function asynchronously and change their states at different rates, speeding up and slowing down independently of other subsystems.

Thus if dynamical systems theory is to be useful it will be at best a characterization of relatively low level implementation details of some of the subsystems. It does not provide a useful framework for specifying how intelligent mind-like control systems differ from such things as weather systems.

8. Towards a taxonomy of interacting substates and causal links

In order to make progress with this approach to the study of mind we need to develop a collection of concepts for describing different substates of an intelligent control system. This will be an iterative process, starting with some initial concepts and then refining, discarding or extending them in the light of experience of attempts to survey an increasing variety of designs in increasing depth. In order to start the process, I'll use terms from ordinary language to bootstrap a new conceptual framework. In particular, the following types of substates seem to be important for mind-like control systems:

- *Desire-like* control states: these can be thought of as initiating processes, maintaining or modifying processes, and terminating processes, of various kinds. Some desire-like states create or modify other desire-like substates rather than directly generating or modifying behaviour. Speaking loosely we can say that causation 'flows away' from desire-like states to produce changes elsewhere. George Kiss at the Open University pointed out to me that the concept of 'attractor' in dynamical systems theory, namely a region in phase space towards which a system tends and from which it does not emerge once having entered, is partially like a desire-like state. It seems unlikely to me that this notion of an attractor is general enough to play the role of desire-like control states in intelligent systems. There are several reasons for this, including the fact that some desire-like states appear to have a complex internal structure (e.g. wanting to find or build a house with a certain layout) that does not seem to be capable of being well represented by a region in phase space. Moreover desire-like states can themselves be the objects of internal manipulation, for instance when an agent suppresses a desire, or reasons about conflicting desires in deciding what to do. Of course, in principle a defender of the dynamical systems analysis could try to construe this as a higher level dynamical system with its own attractors operating on a lower level one. Whether this way of looking at things adds anything useful remains to be seen.

- *Belief-like* control states: these are more passive states produced and changed by causes 'flowing into' them. Only in combination with desire-like states will they tend to produce major new processes. (I do not know whether dynamical systems approach can give a convincing account of how belief-like and desire-like states interact.)

- *Imagination-like* control states: these are states that may be very similar in structure to belief-like states, but have a different causal basis and different causal effects. They may be constructed during processes of deciding what to do by exploring possible consequences of different actions. It is not clear which animals can do this!

- *Plan-like* control states: these are states which have pre-determined sequences of events encoded in a form that is able, via an 'interpreter' mechanism to generate processes controlled by the plan. A stored computer program is a special case of this. Research on planning and acting systems in AI has unearthed a wide variety of forms and functions for such states. A more comprehensive, though still inadequate, list of control states apparently required for intelligent agents can be found in Beaudoin and Sloman (1993).

The concepts introduced here have been 'boostrapped' on our ordinary understanding of words like 'desire' and 'belief' in combination with hints at their significance from the design standpoint. This is an unsatisfactory intermediate state in our understanding, to be remedied later when we have a clearer specification of the functional differences between the different sorts of control states. (The definitions will necessarily be mutually recursive in a systems with many feedback loops, a point implicitly acknowledged by Gilbert Ryle in *The concept of mind* insofar as he rejected the kind of behaviourism that defined mental states purely in terms of external stimuli and behaviour.)

The control states listed above are not the only types of states to be found in intelligent agents: they merely indicate the *sorts* of things that might be found in a taxonomy of substates of an intelligent system. For complete specifications of control systems we would need more than a classification of states. We would also need to specify the relationships between states, such as:

- *Kinds of variability*: how subsystems can change makes a large difference to the kinds of roles they can play. Some physical states can change only by varying one or a few quantitative dimensions, e.g. voltage, temperature. Software developers are now accustomed to a much richer variety of types of change, apparently more suitable for the design of intelligent systems: AI in particular has explored systems making use of changes such as the creation or destruction or modification of symbolic structures in the forms of propositions, trees, networks of symbols. Often what determines the suitability of a mechanism for a functional role is whether it can support the right *kind* of variability and at a suitable *speed*. It is difficult for physical mechanisms to change their structure quickly, so the full range of structural variability at high speed may be achievable only in virtual machines rather than physical machines.

- *What 'flows' in causal channels*: In many control systems the nature of the causal link between subsystems can be described in terms of flow of something (e.g. amount of liquid, amount of electric current) or some physical quantity like force, torque or voltage. By contrast in intelligent systems the causal links may often best be described in terms of a flow of information (including questions, requests, goals, instructions, rules and factual information). The information that flows may itself have a complex structure (like the grammatical structure of a sentence) rather than being a measurable quantity.

- *Remoteness and proximity of causal links*: Some causal links between substates are tight and direct links between substates of directly interacting submechanisms, for instance certain reflexes, whereas other links are *loose* and *indirect,* such as the causal links between input and output channels where the interaction is mediated by many other internal states. The causal connection between something like a preference for socialism and actual behaviour (e.g. political canvassing) would typically be extremely indirect and mediated by many mechanisms.

- *Hierarchical control structures*: Some internal control states (e.g. desire-like states) may produce behaviour of a specific kind fairly directly whereas others (e.g. high-level attitudes, ideals, and personality traits) work through a control hierarchy, for instance, by changing other desire-like states rather than directly triggering behaviour. *Figure 1* gives an approximate indication of this. States that are at a high level in the hierarchy may be longer lasting, more resistant to change, more general in their effects, less direct in their effects, less specific in their control of details of behaviour (internal or external). For example a person's generosity is likely to be high level in this sense, unlike a desire to scratch an itch. Some control states are long term dispositions that are hard to change (e.g. personality, attitudes), others more episodic and transient (e.g. desires, beliefs, intentions, moods). Some of the control relationships are very direct: from sensory stimulation to action (as in innate or trained reflexes). Many of the high level states are complex, richly-structured, sub-states, e.g. political attitudes. Causal interactions involving these are both context-sensitive (dispositional) and (in some cases) probabilistic (propensities, tendencies), not deterministic. Engineers know about control hierarchies, but we need richer mechanisms than *parameter adjustment*.
- *Time-sharing* of causal channels: information channels may be shared between different subsystems, and between different purposes or tasks. This point is elaborated below.

These are merely some initial suggestions regarding the conceptual framework within which it may be useful to analyse control systems in general and intelligent control systems in particular. A lot more work needs to be done, including exploration of design requirements, specifications, designs and mechanisms, and analysis of trade-offs between different designs. All this work will drive further development of our concepts.

9. Control system architectures

Systems vary in their underlying *mechanisms* (e.g. chemical, neural, symbolic, digital, analog, etc.), and, more importantly, in their *architectures*. Within a complex architecture with many different compo-

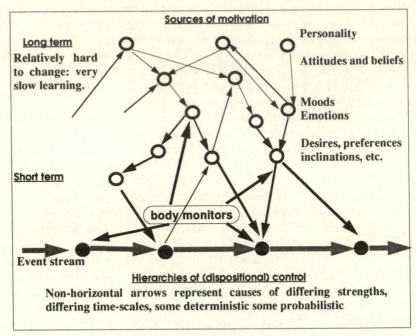

Figure 1

nents different (changeable) control substates may have different functional roles. There is a huge variety of possible architectures for control systems, depending on the number and variety of types of components, types of links, types of causal influences, types of variability of components, and the number and variety of higher level feedback loops implemented by the architecture. One way of beginning to understand the dimensions of variation in control system designs is to examine example systems to see how they can be changed to produce different systems with different capabilities. A full survey would be many lifetimes' work, but we can get some idea of what is involved by looking at some special cases.

Thermostats provide a very simple illustration of the idea that a control system can include substates with different functional roles. A thermostat typically has two control states, one *belief-like* (B1) set by the temperature sensor and one *desire-like* (D1), set by the control knob (*Figure 2*).

- B1 tends to be modified by changes in a feature of the environment E1 (its temperature), using an appropriate sensor (S1), e.g. a bi-metallic strip.
- D1 tends, in combination with B1, to produce changes in E1, via an appropriate output channel (O1)) (I've omitted the heater or

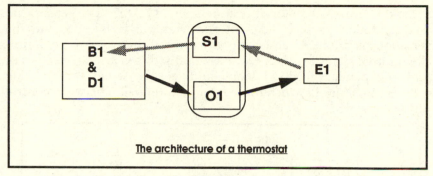

The architecture of a thermostat

Figure 2

cooler.) This is a particularly simple feedback control loop: The states (D1 and B1) both admit one-dimensional continuous variation. D1 is changed by 'users', e.g. via a knob or slider, not shown in this loop.

Arguing whether a thermostat *really* has desires is silly: the point is that it has different coexisting substates with different functional roles, and the terms 'belief-like' and 'desire-like' are merely provisional labels for those differences, until we have a better collection of theory-based concepts. More complex control systems have a far greater variety of coexisting substates. We need to understand that variety. Thermostats are but a simple limiting case. In particular they have no mechanisms for changing their own desire-like states, and there is no way in which their belief-like states can include errors which they can detect, unlike a computer which, for example, can create a structure in one part of its memory summarizing the state of another part: the summary can get out of date and the computer may need to check from time to time by examining the second portion of memory, and updating the summary description if necessary. By contrast the thermostat includes a device that directly registers temperature: There is no check. A more subtle type of thermostat could learn to predict changes in temperature. It would check its predictions and modify the prediction algorithm from time to time, as neural nets and other AI learning systems do.

Moving through design-space we find architectures that differ from the thermostat in the kinds of sub-states, the number and variety of sub-states, the functional differentiation of sub-states, and the kinds of causal influences on substates, such as whether the machine can change its own desire-like states.

Systems with more complex architectures can simultaneously control several different aspects of the environment. For example, *Figure 3* represents a system involving three independently variable states of the environment, E1, E2, E3, sensed using sensors S1, S2,

S3, and altered using output channels: O1, O2, O3. The sensors are causally linked to belief-like internal states, B1, B2, B3, and the behaviour is produced under the influence of these and three desire-like internal states D1, D2, D3. Essentially this is just a collection of three independent feedback loops, and, as such, is not as interesting as an architecture in which there is more interaction between control subsystems.

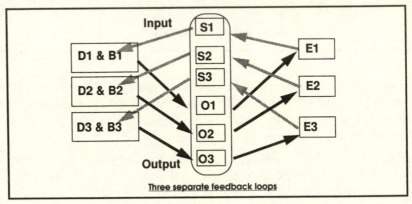

Figure 3

The architecture can be more complicated in various ways: e.g. sharing channels, using multiple layers of input or output processing, self monitoring, self-modification, etc. Some of these complications will now be illustrated.

An interesting constraint that can force internal architectural complexity occurs in many biological systems and some engineering systems: Instead of having separate sensors (Si) and output channels (Oi) for each environmental property, belief-like and desire-like state (Ei, Bi, Di) a complex system might share a collection of Si and Oi between different sets of Ei, Bi, Di, as shown in *Figure 4*. The sharing may be either simultaneous (with data relevant to two tasks superimposed) or successive.

Examples of shared input and output channels are:

- Sharing two eyes (S1, S2) between a collection of beliefs about different bits of the environment
- Sharing two hands (O1, O2) between different desires relating to the state of the environment, for instance pushing a door open whilst carrying a bulky object.
- Sharing large numbers of retinal cells and millions of visual pathways between processes of perception of several different objects simultaneously visible in the environment.
- Sharing millions of motor pathways among a smaller collection of tasks involving manipulating objects in the environment.

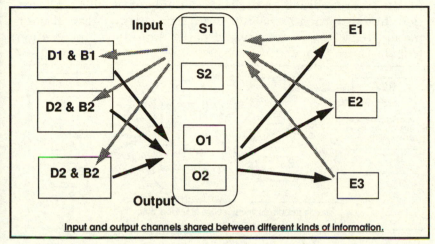

Input and output channels shared between different kinds of information.

Figure 4

- Time-sharing input or output channels between different perceptual processes or different actions done in sequence. For instance first looking in one direction then in another direction, or first carrying one thing then another.

The need to decode information distributed over multiple sensory input channels, and the need to be able to compose control signals to produce co-ordinated contractions in many muscles in order to achieve a common goal are both requirements that lead to quite complex internal information processing. These may have been among the factors driving the evolutionary development of animal brains. Some of these points will now be illustrated in a little more detail.

10. Multi-layered bi-directional sensory processing

Production of belief-like states from sensory information can be more complicated than the examples presented so far.

- Sharing input channels between different Ei and Bi necessitates *interpretation* processes, to extract information relevant to different Bi from sensory 'arrays.' Often this requires specialized knowledge to play a role: general principles do not suffice for disambiguation. E.g. getting 3-D structure from 2-D visual arrays is a mathematically indeterminate problem, yet human brains solve it very rapidly. For this reason, and for the sake of speed, or coping with noisy signals, some or all of the Bi may be produced or modified on the basis not only of *incoming* information, but also using *previously stored* particular or general information (e.g. knowledge-driven, partly 'top-down' perception) (*Figure 5*).

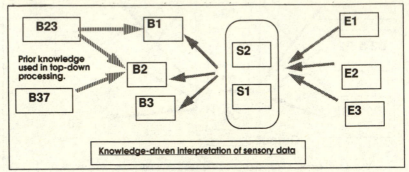

Figure 5

- *Many layers of interpretation may be needed*: Sometimes it is impossible to extract information about the environment in one step. Different intermediate processes may be required, each producing different kinds of data, which may then be combined in the process of arriving at a single high level interpretation. For different purposes, different depths of processing of incoming information may be required, as shown in *Figure 6* (E.g. phonemes, words, phrases, meanings, theories.)

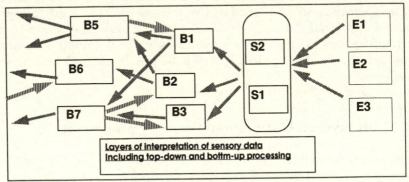

Figure 6

- In some cases the multi-layered processes may also include 'top-down' flow, with partial results in intermediate information stores used partly to control further processing at lower levels (nearer the sensory periphery). This is an example of an internal feedback control loop.

- Different layers of interpretation may use different forms of information storage: retino-topic, analogical, histograms, 'structural descriptions' (e.g. trees, networks), labels for recognized complexes, etc. Whether there is any single good general purpose shape representation is an unsolved problem in AI. It may be that very specific mechanisms are required for creating visual percepts at different levels of interpretation (see *Figure* 7 Section 11).

- Different intermediate 'databases' may be used for different purposes (e.g. some intermediate visual information stores are used, unconsciously, for posture control as well as contributing to perception and recognition of objects in the environment). These different uses may need different 'inference' mechanisms as well as different representational systems.

- Some of the Bi may be stored for future use, or may modify previous long term information stores. Some Bi will be generalizations derived from many particular Bi. Some may be highly tuned specialisations derived from more general forms.

- *Internal self monitoring is possible*: some control loops involve only *internal* processes and substates, like a thermostat whose E1 is part of the internal virtual machine, not a property of the physical environment. An example is a computer operating system that keeps track of how much swapping and paging it does, or which builds internal summaries of some of its own internal structures, which it can also change, like building an index to a database. The development of internal self monitoring and self control submechanisms may be one of the factors that ultimately produced what we think of as human (self) consciousness, though this is a very muddled and ill-defined notion.

- Time-sharing of input channels may require inputs received at *different times* to be integrated for certain of the Bi (e.g. looking at different parts of a house in order to grasp its structure). This requires temporary information stores that can continue to hold information after the sensory input has ended. There may be different information stores at different levels of processing, with different time delays.

All of these points have implications for the architecture (the global design) of a perceiving agent. But we still understand very little about what the full requirements are for human-like perceptual processing, nor what kinds of designs are capable of meeting those requirements, nor what the trade-offs are between different solutions.

11. An example: perceptual architectures

Perception does not merely label things. Visual functions also include providing explanations ('that's how the clock works'), controlling actions (e.g. fine-grained control of movements) and many inner reflexes (e.g. being reminded, finding something or someone beautiful or repulsive). The sort of architecture that seems to be required in a visual system with these diverse capabilities illustrates many of the points already made. For example, a visual system typically (though not necessarily) includes retinal images (which are strictly themselves only rapidly changing samples of the less rapidly changing available 'optic array', as J. J. Gibson (1979) put it). In addition there appear to be requirements for several very different intermediate databases of information derived from a combination of retinal input and, when appropriate, other information. Examples of such intermediate databases are:

- Edge-maps, texture-maps, colour maps, intensity maps, optical flow maps, etc.
- Histograms of various sorts (Hough transforms)
- Databases of edges, lines, regions, binocular disparities, specularities (highlights), colour, etc.
- Groupings into larger 2-D substructures, recognizable 2-D objects, descriptions of their relationships (e.g. near to or overlapping in the visual field, relative size, etc.)
- Databases of 3-D shape fragments inferred from:
  - intensity and colour variation
  - optical flow
  - texture
  - stereo (binocular disparities)
  - edge contour information
- Groupings into larger 3-D substructures (e.g. surfaces, corners, limbs, eyes)
- Descriptions of 3-D shapes of visible objects, and their spatial, causal and functional relationships in the scene, and processes involving them:
  - spatial (inside, next to, touching . . .)
  - causal (pushing, pulling, pressing, twisting)
  - functional (part of, holding up, keeping shut, guiding)
  - intentional (walking towards, picking up, etc.)
- Names of types of things that have been recognized: e.g. a particular combination of 3-D surfaces, edges, corners, etc. may be recognized as a table, and another as a chair. Some recognition may be based on 2-D structures. Some names will label recognized actions, e.g. a pirouette, opening a door, pouring a liquid, etc.

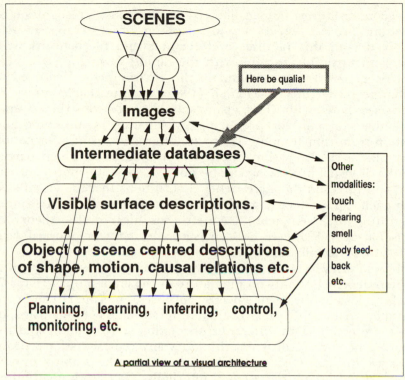

Figure 7

Figure 7 is an attempt to illustrate all this architectural richness in a visual system, albeit in a very sketchy fashion.

In human beings some, but not all, of the intermediate perceptual information stores are accessible to internal self-monitoring processes, e.g. for the purpose of reporting how things look (as opposed to how they are), or painting scenes, or controlling actions on the basis of visible relationships in the 2-D visual field. I believe that this is the source of the kinds of experiences that make some philosophers wish to talk about 'qualia'. From this viewpoint, qualia, rather than being hard to accommodate in mechanistic or functional terms, exist as an *inevitable* consequence of perceptual design requirements. Of course, there are philosophers who add additional requirements to qualia that make them incapable of being explained in this way: but I suspect that those additional requirements also make qualia figments of such philosophers' imaginations. Not pure figments, since such philosophical tendencies are a result of the existence of real qualia of the sort described here.

Vision, or at least human-like vision, is not just a recognition or labelling process: creation and mapping of structures is also involved, and this requires architectures and mechanisms with sufficient flexibility to cope with the rapidly changing structures that occur as we move around in the environment. I've tried to elaborate on all this in Sloman (1989) arguing that contrary to views associated with Marr, vision should not be construed simply as being a system for producing information about shape and motion from retinal input. There are other sources of information that play a role in vision, there are other uses to which partial results of visual processing can be put (e.g. posture control, attention control), and there are richer descriptions that the visual system itself can produce (e.g. when a face looks happy, sad, dejected, beautiful, intelligent, etc.) Dennett's 'multiple drafts' theory of consciousness (1991) can be seen as a somewhat metaphorical variant of these design ideas from AI.

The internal information structures produced by a perceptual system depend not only on the nature of the environment (E1, E2, etc.) but also on the agent's needs, purposes, etc. (the Di) and conceptual apparatus. Because of this, different kinds of organisms, or even two people with different information stores, can look at the same scene and see different things. Many representational problems are still unsolved, including, for instance the problem of how arbitrary shapes are represented internally. Clues to human information structures and processes come from analysing examples in great detail, such as examples of things we can see, how they affect us, and what we can do as a result. I believe that every aspect of human experience is amenable to this kind of functional analysis, and that supposed counter-examples are put forward only because many philosophers do not have sufficient design creativity: most of them are not good cognitive engineers!

12. Kinds of variability in perceived structures

Different mechanisms (or parts of one mechanism) provide different kinds of variation. A temperature sensor requires only *linear* (continuous?) variation. A house-perceiver or sentence-understander needs *structural* variation. *Figure 8* illustrates some of the ways visual percepts can change in structure. The changes may be purely geometric or they may be more abstract and subtle, as when the duck-rabbit flips. Exactly what sorts of internal variability are required for different sub-mechanisms is still not understood, nor which mechanisms are capable of supporting which kinds of variability.

For example, it may be that variations during construction of a

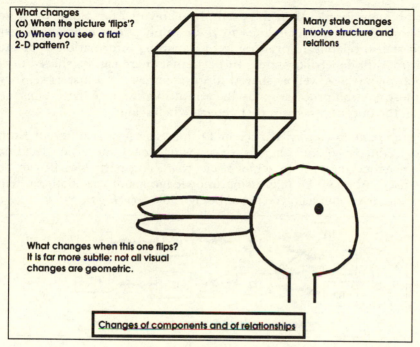

Figure 8

plan of action, variations during visual perception of a continuously moving object, and variations when wondering what conclusions can be drawn from some puzzling evidence all require very different internal structural changes, and that different sorts of sub-mechanisms are therefore required.

The kind of variability needed in Bi and Di states depends on both the environment (e.g. does it contain things with different structures, things with changing structures, etc.?) and the requirements and abilities of the agent. Compare the needs of a fly and of a person. Do flies need to see structures (e.g. for mating)? Do they deliberately create or modify structures? Rivers don't. There is lots more work to be done analysing the design requirements for various organisms in terms of their functional requirements in coping with the environment and with each other. This is one way in which to provide a conceptual framework for investigating the evolution of mind-like capabilities of different degrees of sophistication.

13. Architectural variety regarding desire-like sub-states

There are various ways in which the generation of outputs from desire-like states (in combination with belief-like states) may be more complicated than the examples shown so far. Some of these complications are analogous to the complications previously discussed in relation to processing of incoming information to create or modify belief-like states. In particular there can be shared output channels as well as shared input channels, and just as sensory interpretation processes may have multiple intermediate states, so can the output processes that generate behaviour.

- *Information sharing*: Particular Di may use several different Bi in producing output signals (e.g. using many facts in deciding whether and how to achieve one goal), and particular Bi can be used by many Di (e.g. using knowledge about cars both to help you drive, and help you avoid being run over) (*Figure 9*).

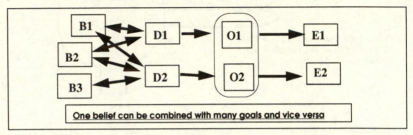

One belief can be combined with many goals and vice versa

Figure 9

- Causal links between Di and Oi may be indirect, via several layers of causation (*Figure 10*), e.g.
  (a) going via planning mechanisms, and using different sub-goals to achieve a single goal
  (b) translating high-level to low-level instructions.

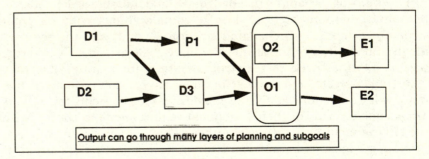

Output can go through many layers of planning and subgoals

Figure 10

- Just as there is internal monitoring so can there be internal behaviour. Some Di change internal states, e.g. other Di and Bi. So some control is *self* control: e.g. making yourself concentrate on something. In that case some of the Ei are internal (the mind is part of the environment, for itself). Desires themselves may be produced by deeper or higher level desire-like states (e.g. general attitudes, preferences, etc.) interacting with various Bi to produce new motives. So motivation can involve *hierarchies* of dispositions. (see *Figure 1*).

- Some Di are long term *dispositions* to produce various changes: they don't actually *do* anything until certain conditions arise, e.g. personality traits, and attitudes like racial prejudice. (Compare the previous comments on hierarchies of dispositional control states.)
- Some 'higher level' control states will not be concerned with particular goals or desires, but with principles or preferences for selecting between conflicting Di.
- Different intermediate Di-controlled sub-states in 'output' pathways may use different forms of information storage and transmission, (compare layers of interpretation of inputs), e.g. having a thought, shaping a sentence, generating a syntactic form, selecting words, intonation patterns, stress patterns, volume, etc. may all require different intermediate data representations. Compare dancing, sculpting, assembling a clock.
- The Di need not determine *instantaneous* output: they may require *temporally extended* actions. This requires
  (a) Di states with rich internal structure (e.g. stored plans, with suitable temporary memory mechanisms)
  (b) 'output channels' with considerable sophistication (e.g. program-execution mechanism for 'translating' static plans into behaviour in time, rule-following mechanisms, etc.)
- In a system that is required to control continuous physical movement, it is likely that some of the output signals are not discrete instructions to 'motors' to perform complete steps. Instead there may be continuously varying output signals, such as a voltage or torque, whilst the effects of the behaviour thus produced are monitored continuously and the results used to modify the output: i.e. there are some continuous feedback control loops. An example would be the fine-grained control of motion of a violin bow so as to produce a sustained beautiful tone. Other cases may include a mixture of continuous and discrete monitoring and control, e.g. looking where you are walking, to make sure you are still on the intended route to your destination. A discrete high level signal could be an instruction to turn left at a certain corner. At lower levels control might still be continuous.
- The global control architecture itself may need to change as a result of learning. For example, number and variety of Bi and

Di (and other types of control sub-states) change over time, and new causal linkages develop:
- A child eventually learns not to let the latest powerful motive dominate. What architectural changes enable the developing child to compare different motives, assess short and long term benefits?
- Some of the structures, and structural changes produced by the control processes, like changes in the Bi, may occur only in high level *virtual* machines.

14. What sorts of underlying mechanisms are needed?

The discussion so far is neutral as to what physical mechanisms are used to implement the various kinds of substates and causal linkages. They might be neural mechanisms or some other kind. As in circuit design, the global properties of the architecture are more important than which particular mechanisms are used, when the overall design is right.

Architecture dominates mechanism

The detailed mechanisms make only marginal differences as long as they support the design features required for reasons given earlier, such as:

- sufficient structural variability
- sufficient architectural richness
  - number of independently variable components
  - functional differentiation of components
  - variety of causal linkages
- sufficient speed of operation
- sufficiently smooth performance for controlling physical movement.

As we've argued above, 'virtual' machines in computers seem to have some of the required features, including rich structural variability and the ability to change structures very quickly. It may be that brains can also do this, though if they do it will also most likely involve another virtual mechanism, for it is not possible for networks of nerve cells to change their structures rapidly. In computers the virtual machine structures are usually implemented in terms of changing configurations of bit patterns in memory. Perhaps in brains it is done via changing configurations of activation patterns of neurones. In computers the same mechanisms are used for both short term and long term changes (except where long term changes are copied into a slower less volatile memory medium such as magnetic disks and tapes). In brains it seems likely that different mechanisms are used for long term and short term changes. For example in some neural net models the long term changes require changing 'weights' on excitatory and inhibitory links between neurones, and getting these changes to occur seems to require much longer 'training' processes than the changing patterns of activation produced by new neural inputs. (However, there are well known remembering tricks that produce 'one shot' long term learning.) It seems very likely that there are other kinds of important processes used in brains including chemical processes.

Whatever the actual biological implementation mechanisms may be it is at least theoretically possible that the very same functional architectures are capable of being implemented in different low-level mechanisms. It is equally possible that this is ruled out in our physical world because some of the processes require tight coupling between high level and low level machines, and it could turn out that in our universe the only way to achieve this is to use a particular type of brain-like implementation. For example, it could turn out that, in our universe, *only* a mixture of electrical pathways and chemical soup could provide the right combination of fine-grained control, structural variability and global control. I have no reason to believe that there is such a restriction on possible implementations: I merely point out that it is a possibility that should not be ruled out at this stage.

But we don't know enough about requirements, nor about available mechanisms, to really say yet which infrastructure could and which couldn't work These are issues still requiring research (not philosophical pontificating!).

15. The shape of design space

I've suggested earlier that it is not enough to produce a single design: in order to understand the costs and benefits of particular designs we need to explore alternative designs in order to understand how they differ in the kinds of behaviours they support and their implementation requirements. Within the framework of such a design-based theory we may be better able to formulate sensible questions about how behavioural capabilities evolved in biological organisms, and instead of being faced with unanswerable questions such as 'Which animals are and which are not conscious?' we can hope to use new technical concepts for classifying natural and artificial behaving systems.

Many people feel that their concepts are so clear and precise that they can be used to produce a sharp division in the world, i.e. there is a major dichotomy like that shown in *Figure 11*. Unfortunately,

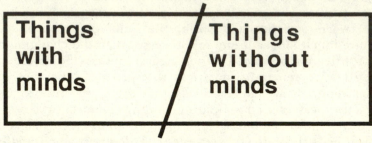

Figure 11

when they attempt to decide where the dividing line actually is they generally find it so hard to provide one, especially one on which everyone will agree, that many of them then jump to the conclusion that the space is a smooth continuum with no natural division, so that it's a purely a matter of convenience where the line should be drawn. So they think of design space like *Figure 12*.

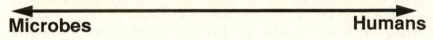

Figure 12

This is a deep mistake: any software designer will appreciate that there are *many* important discontinuities in designs. For instance a multi-branch conditional instruction in a typical programming language can have 10 branches or 11 branches but cannot have 10.5 or 10.25 or 10.125 branches. Each condition-action pair is either present or not present.

Similarly, a machine can have skids for moving over the ground or it can have wheels, but there is no continuous set of transformations that will gradually transform a skidded vehicle to a wheeled vehicle: eventually there will be a discontinuity when the system changes from being made of one piece to being made of pieces that can move against each other (like an axle in a hole). If we think of biological organisms as forming a continuum then we fail to notice that there is a very important research task to be done, namely to explore the *many* design discontinuities in order to understand where they occur, what difference it makes to an organism whether it is on one side or the other of the discontinuity, and what kinds of evolutionary pressures might have supported the discontinuous jump. (Notice that none of this is an argument in support of a creationist metaphysics: it is a direct consequence of Darwinian theory that since acquired characteristics cannot be inherited there can only be a finite number of designs occurring between any two points in time, and therefore there must be many discontinuous changes, even if many of them are small discontinuities, such as going from N to N+1 components where N is already large.)

However it could well turn out that some of the discontinuities were of major significance. So we should keep an open mind and, for the time being, assume that design space includes a large number of discontinuities of varying significance, some far more important than others. We could picture it something like *Figure 13*. This picture is still too simple: e.g. it is single-layered, whereas different maps may required for different levels of design. There are still many design options and trade-offs that we don't yet understand. We need a whole family of new concepts, based on a theory of *design architectures and mechanisms*, to help us understand the relation between structure and capability (form and function).

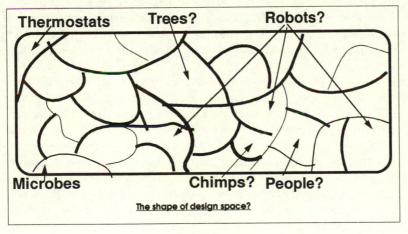

Figure 13

16. Towards a general theory of attention

One implication of the kind of architecture sketched above is that there are typically multiple causal channels between sub-mechanisms. Thus any event or process occurring at one part of the system may have different effects elsewhere depending on which interactions are allowed to happen. This implies a need for many kinds of internal control in order to determine which causal channels are allowed to operate: which kinds of information are allowed to go to which sub-systems, and what is done with them. One example is deciding which subset of current sensory input should be processed and how it should be processed. Another example is deciding which current goals should be acted on and how they should be acted on.

Within this framework we can construe different kinds of attention in terms of different ways patterns of activity can be selected. The selection may involve changing which information is analysed, how it is analysed (i.e. which procedures are applied), and selecting where the results should go. Another example would be selecting which goals to think about or act on, and, for selected goals, choosing between alternative issues to address, e.g. choosing between working out whether to adopt or reject the goal, working out how urgent or important it is, selecting or creating a plan for achieving it, etc.

Some selections will be based solely on what is desirable to the system or serves its needs. However, sometimes two or more activities that are both desirable cannot both be pursued because they are incompatible, such as requiring the agent to be in two places at once, or looking in two directions at once or requiring more simultaneous internal processing than the agent is capable of. The precise reasons why human thought processes are resource limited is not clear, but resource limited they certainly are. So the control of attention is important, and allowing control to be lost and attention to be diverted can sometimes be disastrous. The architecture should therefore include mechanisms that have the ability to filter out attention distractors.

These remarks are typical of the problems that arise when one adopts the design stance that would not normally occur to philosophers who don't do so. Their significance is that they point to the need for mechanisms in realistic, resource-limited, agents in terms of which mental states and processes can be defined that would be totally irrelevant to idealised agents that had unlimited processing capabilities and storage space. Thus, in so far as it is part of the job of philosophers to analyse concepts that we use for describing the mental states and processes of real agents, and not just hypothetical imaginary ideal agents, philosophers need to adopt the design stance.

This can be illustrated with the example of a certain kind of emotional state. I have tried to show elsewhere (Sloman and Croucher 1981, Sloman1987, Beaudoin and Sloman 1993) that certain kinds of resource-limited systems can get into states that have properties closely related to familiar aspects of certain emotional states, namely those in which there is a partial loss of control of our own thought processes. I call these states *perturbances*. Such capabilities would not be the product of specific mechanisms for producing those states, but would be *emergent* properties of sophisticated resource-limited control systems, just as saltiness emerges when chlorine and sodium combine, and 'thrashing' can emerge in an overloaded computer operating system. Our vocabulary for describing such emergent global states will improve with increased understanding of the underlying mechanisms.

There are many shallow views about emotional states, including the view that they are essentially concerned with experience of physiological processes. If that were true then anaesthetizing the body would be a way to remove grief over the death of a loved one.

A deeper analysis shows, I believe, that what is important to the grieving mother (and those who are close to her) is that she can't help thinking back about the lost child, and what she might have done to prevent the death, and what would have happened if the child had lived on, etc. There may also be physiological processes and corresponding sensory feedback but in the case of grief they are of secondary importance. The socially and personally important aspects of grief (i.e. perturbances) are closer to control states of a sophisticated information processing system.

Several AI groups are now beginning to explore these issues. But there is much that we still don't understand about design requirements relating to the sources of motivation and the kinds of processes that can occur in a system with its own motivational substates.

17. Further implications

Although the ideas sketched here do not constitute a full blown theory, but merely indicate the outlines of a research programme, I believe they have many deep implications for old philosophical problems about the nature of mind, the relations between mind and body, and the analysis of mental concepts. I shall conclude by drawing attention to an arbitrarily selected subset of these implications.

It is often said that a machine could never have any goals of its own: all of its goals would essentially be goals of the programmer or the 'user.' However, consider a machine that has the kind of hierarchy of dispositional control states described previously, analogous to very general traits, more specific but still general attitudes, preferences, and specific desire-like states. Now suppose that it also includes 'learning' mechanisms such that the states at all levels in the hierarchy are capable of being modified as a result of a long history of interaction with the environment, including other agents. After a long period of interacting with other agents and modifying itself at different levels in the control hierarchy such a machine might respond to a new situation by generating a particular goal. The processes producing that goal could not be attributed entirely to the designer. In fact, there will be such a multiplicity of causes that there may not be any candidate for 'ownership' of the new goal other than the machine itself. This, it seems to me, is no different from the situation with regard to human motives which likewise come from a rich and complex interplay of genetic mechanisms, parental influences and short and long term, direct and indirect effects of interaction with the individual's environment, including absorption of a culture.

Issues concerning 'freedom of the will' get solved or dissolved by analysing types and degrees of autonomy within systems so designed, so that the free/unfree dichotomy disappears (compare Dennett 1984, Sloman 1978).

Exploration of important discontinuities in design-space could lead to the formulation of important new questions about when and how these discontinuities occurred in biological evolution. For example, it could turn out that the development of a hierarchy of dispositional control states was a major change from simpler mechanisms permitting only one control loop to be active at a time. Another discontinuity might have been the development of the ability to defer some goals and re-invoke them later on: that requires a more complex storage architecture than a system that always has only one 'adopted' goal at a time. Perhaps the ability to cope with rapid *structural* variation in information stores was another major evolutionary advance in biological control systems, probably requiring the use of virtual machines.

One implication of the claim that there's not just one major discontinuity, but a large collection of different discontinuities of varying significance is that many of our concepts that are normally used as if there were a dichotomy cannot be used to formulate meaningful questions of the form 'Which organisms have X and which organisms don't?', 'How did X evolve?' 'What is the biological function of X?' This point can be made about a variety of substitutes for X, e.g. 'consciousness', 'intelligence', 'intentionality', 'rationality', 'emotions' and others.

However, a systematic exploration of the possibilities in design space could lead us to replace the supposed monolithic concepts with collections of different concepts corresponding to different combinations of capabilities. Detailed analysis of the functional differentiation of substates and the varieties of process that are possible could produce a revised vocabulary for kinds of mental states and process. Thus, instead of the one ill-defined concept 'consciousness' we might find it useful to define a collection of theoretically justified precisely defined concepts C1, C2, C3 . . . Cn, which can be used to ask scientifically answerable questions of the above forms.

This evolution of a new conceptual framework for talking about mental states and processes could be compared with the way early notions of kinds of stuff were replaced by modern scientific concepts as a result of the development of the atomic theory of matter.

18. The richness and inaccessibility of internal states and processes

One feature of the kind of architecture outlined here is that there are large numbers of active internal causal pathways, with many internal feedback loops. This makes the whole system inherently unstable: internal states are constantly in flux, even without external stimulation. Most of the 'behaviour' of such a machine would then be internal (including changes within virtual machines). Moreover, since most of the causal relationships between external stimuli and subsequent behaviour in such a system would be mediated by *internal* states, and since these states are in a state of flux, the chance of finding interesting correlations between external stimuli and responses would be very low, making the task of experimental psychology almost hopelessly difficult except, perhaps, with regard to peripheral and certain global processes.

For similar reasons, there would not necessarily be any close correspondence between internal control states such as the Bi and Di, and external circumstances and behaviour. So, for such a system, inferring inner states from behaviour with any reliability is nearly impossible. Moreover, if many of the important control states are states in virtual machines there won't be much hope of checking them out by opening up the machine and observing the internal physical states either. This provides a kind of scientific justification for philosophical scepticism about other minds.

Thus, even if design-based studies lead to the development of a new systematic collection of concepts for classifying types of mental states and processes it may be very difficult to apply those concepts to particular cases. This could be put in the form of a paradox: *by taking the design stance seriously we can produce reasons why the design stance is almost impossible to apply to the understanding of particular individuals which we have not designed ourselves.*

If some of the internal processes are 'self-monitoring' processes that produce explicit summary descriptions of what's going on (inner percepts?) these could give the agent the impression of full awareness of his own internal states. But if the self-monitoring processes are selective and geared to producing only information that is of practical use to the system, then it will no more give complete and accurate information about internal states and processes than external perceptual processes give full and accurate information about the structure of matter. Thus the impression of perfect self-knowledge will be an illusion. Nevertheless the fact that all this happens could be what explains the strong temptation to talk about 'qualia' felt by many philosophers. I have previously drawn attention to the special case of this where internal monitoring processes can access intermediate visual databases.

More generally, a host of notions involving sentience, self-monitoring capabilities, high-level control of internal and external processes including attention, and the ability to direct attention internally, including attending to 'qualia', could all be accounted for by a suitable information-processing control system.

19. Potential practical implications

The new conceptual framework could be of great practical importance in connection with improving the human lot. Human mental processes often seem to go wrong, for example multiple personalities, emotional disorders, learning disabilities. This is not at all surprising in such a complex system. In fact it is hard to understand how coherent control of such a system is possible at all, and why it doesn't go wrong more often. When things do go wrong, you can't hope to be much good at helping (therapy, counselling, training) without knowing the underlying design principles. Otherwise it's a hit and miss affair (i.e. craft, not science or engineering. But some 'craft' skills are highly effective, even if we don't know why!).

When we have a good design-based theory of how complex human-like systems work it could lead us to many new insights concerning ways in which they can go wrong. This could, for example, help us to design improved teaching and learning strategies, and strategies for helping people with emotional and other problems. If we acquire a better understanding of mechanisms underlying learning, motivation, emotions, etc. then perhaps we can vastly improve procedures in education, psychotherapy, counselling, and teaching psychologists about how minds work (as opposed to teaching them how to do experiments and apply statistics).

20. Intentionality and semantics

An issue that I have not yet addressed, but which exercises many philosophers, is how semantics can get into the system. What features of the design of a system make it possible for a machine to use one object to represent another? Which organisms are capable of having intentional states in which they somehow refer to objects, and why can't other organisms do it?

By now readers will be aware that such questions are based on the unjustified assumption that we have a precisely defined concept which generates a dichotomous division. This is an illusion, just like all the other illusions that bedevil philosophical discussions about mind. It's an illusion because our ability to represent or think about things is not a monolithic ability which is either entirely absent or all present in every other organism or machine. Rather it's a complex collection of (ill-understood) capabilities different subsets of which may be present in different designs.

One group of relevant capabilities involves the availability of sub-mechanisms with sufficiently varied control states for particular representational purposes. The kinds of variability in the mechanisms required for intermediate visual perception are likely to be quite different from the sorts of variability required for comparing two routes, or thinking about what to do next week. There are probably far more organisms that share with us the former mechanisms than share the latter. We can label the structural richness requirement a *syntactic* requirement.

Another group of requirements involves *functional* diversity of uses of the representing structures. Humans can have states in which they perceive things, wonder about things (e.g. is someone in the next room?), desire things (e.g. wanting a person to accept one's marriage proposal) or plan sequences of actions. Being able to put information structures to all these diverse uses requires an architecture that supports differentiation of roles of sub-mechanisms. Some organisms will have only a small subset of that diversity in common with us, others a larger set. A bird may be capable of perceiving that there are peanuts in a dispenser in the garden, but be incapable of wondering whether there are peanuts in the dispenser or forming the intention to get peanuts into the dispenser. (Of course, I am speaking loosely in saying what it can see: its conceptual apparatus may store information in a form that is not translatable into English. It's hard enough to translate other human languages into English!)

What exactly are the syntactic and functional requirements for full human-like intentionality, i.e. representational capability? I don't yet know: that's another problem on which there's work to be done, though I've started listing some of the requirements in previous papers (Sloman 1985, 1986). One thing that's clear is that any adequate theory of how X can use Y to refer to Z is going to have to cope with far more varied syntactic forms than philosophers and logicians normally consider: besides sentential or propositional forms there will be all the kinds of representing structures that are used in intermediate stages of sensory processing. Thus an adequate theory of semantics must account for the use of pictorial structures and possibly also more abstract representational structures such as patterns of weights or patterns of activation in a neural net.

What convinces me that the problems of filling in the story are not insuperable is the fact that there are clearly primitive semantic capabilities in even the simplest computers, for they can use bit patterns to refer to locations in their memories, or to represent instructions, and they can use more complex 'virtual' structures to represent all sorts of things about their own internal states, including instructions to be obeyed, descriptions of some of their memory contents, and records of their previous behaviour. A machine can even refer to a non-existent portion of its memory if it constructs an 'address' that goes beyond the size of its memory. With more complex architectures they will have richer, more diverse semantic capabilities.

Being able to refer to things outside itself, or even to non-existent things like the person wrongly supposed to be in the next room or the action planned for tomorrow which never materialises, requires the machine to have a systematic and *generative* way of relating internal states to external actual and possible entities, events, processes, etc. Although this may seem difficult in theory, in practice fragmentary versions of such capabilities are already possessed by robots, plant control systems and other computing systems that act semi-autonomously in the world (Sloman 1985,1986). Of course, they don't yet have either the syntactic richness or the functional variety of human representational capabilities, but the question how to extend their capabilities is to be treated as an engineering design problem. Instead of proving that something is or is not possible, philosophical engineers, or design-oriented philosophers, should expect to find a range of options with different strengths and weaknesses.

Anyone who tries to prove that it is impossible to create a machine with semantic capabilities risks joining the ranks of those who 'knew' that the earth was flat, that action at a distance was impossible, that space satisfied Euclidean axioms, that no uncaused events can occur, or that a deity created the universe a few thousand years ago.

References

Beaudoin L. P. and Sloman A.1993, 'A study of motive processing and attention', in A. Sloman, D. Hogg, G. Humphreys, D. Partridge, A. Ramsay (eds) *Prospects for Artificial Intelligence*. Amsterdam, IOS Press.

Dennett D. C. 1978. *Brainstorms: Philosophical Essays on Mind and Psychology*. Harvester Press, Hassocks.

Dennett D. C. 1984 *Elbow Room: The Varieties of Free Will Worth Wanting*. Oxford: Clarendon Press.

Dennett, D. C. 1991. *Consciousness Explained*, Allen Lane, The Penguin Press.

Gibson J. J. 1979. *The Ecological Approach to Visual Perception*. Lawrence Earlbaum Associates (reprinted 1986)

Ryle G. 1949. *The Concept of Mind*. London: Hutchinson.

Searle J. R. 1980 'Minds brains and programs' *The Behavioral and Brain Sciences*, **3**.

Sloman A. 1978. *The Computer Revolution in Philosophy: Philosophy Science and Models of Mind*. Hassocks Harvester Press and Humanities Press.

Sloman A. and Croucher M. 1981. 'Why robots will have emotions', in *Proceedings 7th International Joint Conference on Artificial Intelligence*, Vancouver, also available as Cognitive Science Research Paper 176, Sussex University.

Sloman A. 1985. 'What enables a machine to understand?' in *Proceedings 9th International Joint Conference on AI*, Los Angeles, pp. 995–1001. Also available as Cognitive Science Research Paper 053, Sussex University.

Sloman A. 1986. 'Reference without causal links' in *Proceedings 7th European Conference on Artificial Intelligence*, published as J. B. H. du Boulay, D. Hogg, L. Steels (eds) *Advances in Artificial Intelligence—II* pp. 369–81. North Holland, 1987. Also available as Cognitive Science Research Paper 047, Sussex University

Sloman A. 1987. 'Motives Mechanisms Emotions', *Cognition and Emotion* 1, 3, pp. 217–234, reprinted in M. A. Boden (ed.) *The Philosophy of Artificial Intelligence*, 'Oxford Readings in Philosophy' Series Oxford University Press, pp. 231– 247, 1990.

Sloman A. 1989. 'On designing a visual system: Towards a Gibsonian computational model of vision', *Journal of Experimental and Theoretical AI* 1,

4, pp. 289–337, also available as Cognitive Science Research Paper 146, Sussex University.

Sloman A. 1992. 'The emperor's real mind: review of Roger Penrose's, *The Emperor's new Mind: Concerning Computers Minds and the Laws of Physics*,' Artificial Intelligence, 56, pp. 355–396, also available as Cognitive Science Research Paper, The University of Birmingham.

Sloman A. 1993. 'Prospects for AI as the general science of intelligence', in A. Sloman, D. Hogg, G. Humphreys, D. Partridge, A. Ramsay (eds) *Prospects for Artificial Intelligence*. Amsterdam: IOS Press.

On the Notions of Specification and Implementation*

ANTONY GALTON

In this paper we consider two key concepts from software engineering—'specification' and 'implementation'—and explore their possible applications outside software engineering to other disciplines, notably the philosophy of action, evolutionary biology, and cognitive science. Throughout, the emphasis is on the gain in conceptual clarity that can be afforded by these concepts; it is not so much a matter of new knowledge or new theories but of a reorganization of existing knowledge and theories in a way that facilitates the transfer of insights across a range of related fields.

The paper begins with an examination of the concepts in their original home of computer science, and then seeks to broaden the perspective by considering, in a general way, how they might find application outside that field. We conclude with three case studies in which we discuss the applicability of the concepts to the description of group action, morphogenesis, and the human mind.

1. Specification and implementation in computer science

In computer science a specification is a more or less precise or exact statement of how a software system is required to behave. It provides a criterion against which the success or correctness of the software system can be judged. Minimally, a specification is a functional specification, that is, it specifies the system as a 'black box' in terms of what output it will deliver when activated by any given input. Nothing is said of, for example, how long it will take to deliver the output, and the specification is pure in the sense that nothing is said about how the generation of output from input is to be achieved.

A very simple example is the problem of sorting a list of words into alphabetical order, which may be specified as follows:

Input: a list of words L_0
Output: an ordered list of words L_1 whose elements are just the elements of L_0.

*This paper has benefited from discussions with Derek Partridge and with Aaron Sloman.

A solution to this problem is an algorithm which contains explicit instructions for deriving output bearing the specified relation to the input. Such an algorithm is called an implementation of the specification. Two solutions to the word-sorting problem are

- **Insertion Sort**. *If L_0 is* nil *(the empty list), set L_1 to be* nil *also. Otherwise L_0 consists of a first word a and a remainder R. Let M be the result of (recursively) sorting R, and then let L_1 be the result of inserting a into its alphabetically correct position in R, where insertion is defined by the following specification:*

   Input: an ordered list of words L_0 and a word a.
   Output: an ordered list of words L_1 whose elements are just the elements of L_0 together with a.

- **Merge Sort**. *If L_0 is* nil*, set L_1 to* nil *also. Otherwise, split L_0 into two parts P_1 and P_2 (so $L_0=P_1+P_2$), and let Q_1 and Q_2 be the results of (recursively) sorting P_1 and P_2 respectively. Let L_1 be the result of merging Q_1 and Q_2, where merging is defined by the specification:*

   Input: two ordered lists of words L_1 and L_2.
   Output: An ordered list of words L whose elements are just the elements of L_1 together with those of L_2.

There are two important things to notice about these implementations. First, they are only partial implementations in that they are not yet completely explicit, they contain terms (namely 'insert' and 'merge') which are only specified, not implemented. Second, a given specification can be implemented in more than one way.

Suppose we remedy the first deficiency by writing down implementations for 'insert' and 'merge', for example:

- Inserting a into ordered list L_0: If L_0 is *nil*, let L_1 be the list whose only member is a. Otherwise, let L_0 consist of the first element b and remainder R. If a is alphabetically earlier than b, let L be the list whose first element is a and whose remainder is L_0; otherwise, let M be the result of (recursively) inserting a into R, and let L_1 be the list whose first element is b and whose remainder is M.

- Merging sorted lists L_1 and L_2: If either L_1 or L_2 is *nil* then set L to be the other one. Otherwise, suppose L_1 and L_2 have first elements a_1 and a_2 respectively and remainders R_1 and R_2. Then if a_1 is alphabetically earlier than a_2, let L be the list whose first element is a_1 and whose remainder is the result of (recursively) merging R_1 with L_2; otherwise let L be the list whose first element is a_2 and whose remainder is the result of merging L_1 with R_2.

We now have two algorithms for sorting a list. According to one usage of the term 'implementation' we have implemented the original specification. On the other hand, people also speak of 'implementing an algorithm'. This means writing a program which can be run on a computer in order to carry out the instructions detailed in the algorithm. This could be done in many different ways: in different programming languages, or using different data structures in the same language. For insertion sort, for example, we could write a Prolog program

```
sort([],[]).
sort([A|R],L) :- sort(R,M), insert(A,M,L).

insert(A,[],[A]).
insert(A,[B|R],[A,B|R]) :- A<B, !.
insert(A,[B|R],[B|M]) :- insert(A,R,M).
```

or a Lisp program

```
(defun sort (1)
  (cond ((null 1) 1)
  (T (insert (car 1) (sort (cdr 1))))))

(defun insert (a 1)
  (cond ((null 1) (list a))
  ((< a (car 1)) (cons a 1))
  (T (cons (car 1) (insert a (cdr 1)))))))
```

These programs are very simple because both Prolog and Lisp have built-in procedures for representing and handling lists; to implement the same algorithm in Pascal one must first decide how one is going to represent the lists (e.g., as arrays, linked lists, or files) and then devise appropriate procedures depending on one's decision.

The point here is that the insertion sort algorithm presented in general terms above does not dictate how one should implement it as a program. It can itself be regarded as a kind of specification, a criterion against which the correctness or otherwise of a program can be judged. If Mary implements the specification of the sorting problem as an algorithm, and Tom then implements her algorithm as a program, and this program doesn't work, that is, it fails to sort correctly the lists it is presented with, then the fault might lie either with Mary or Tom.

But these are not the only possibilities: maybe the compiler, which automatically translates Tom's program into a form that is more directly intelligible to the computer, is at fault; or maybe the design of the computer itself is faulty. One writes a program on the assumption that the programming language itself has been correctly implemented for the type of computer one wishes to use: so lurking in the background there is another specification/implementation relation, which must bridge the gap between the programming language as an abstract medium for the realisation of algorithms and the programming language as an effective means of controlling what actually happens in the computer.

Any component that arises at any stage in the development of a computer system can be viewed in terms of the specification/implementation relation. The notion of correctness has to be understood in a relative way. A program might be proved correct with respect to a formal specification, using the well-known techniques of Hoare, Dijkstra, etc, and this must be interpreted to mean that if the programming language is correctly implemented then the program, when run, will deliver results in accordance with the specification. The 'if' is a big if: implementing the programming language involves writing a compiler or interpreter for it; the definition of the language constitutes, in effect, a specification for a compiler or interpreter of that language, but the implementation of the latter will involve reference to some lower-level implementation technology, and so on down to machine code, microcode, and the hardware itself. At each stage, there is a specification which lays down the behaviour that is required, and the correctness of the implementation at that level only guarantees correct behaviour on the assumption that the lower-level specifications have been correctly implemented. As Fetzer (1988) has pointed out, the notion of mathematical proof can only be applied to the correctness problem at those levels where both the specification and the implementation are well-defined formal objects.

It is normally said that the demand for exact methods of specification and dependable methods of validating implementations against their specifications has arisen because it has been found impossible, without such methods, to produce software that is dependably error-free. On the other hand, it is also suggested that the notion of correctness, and hence of an 'error' in software, has to be understood in relation to an exact specification. But if that is the case, then the story just told cannot be true: if errors only exist in relation to specifications, then it cannot have been the presence of errors that led to the need for specifications in the first place. It follows that the idea of an error (and hence, of correctness) must precede the notion of a specification.

The classic 'software cycle' envisages that first one formalizes one's requirements as a specification, then one produces some software, and then one verifies that the software meets the specification. In practice, as Swartout and Balzer (1983) point out, specification and implementation are 'inevitably intertwined': one modifies the specification in step with one's experience in trying to implement it. This is sometimes reviled as the vice of 'hacking', but the desirability or otherwise of such practice is surely a function of how responsibly and systematically it is pursued. To suppose that one can specify everything in advance is the height of arrogance: we all make mistakes, and the worst thing is to commit oneself to them irrevocably.

At the other extreme there is the idea of a *'post hoc'* specification. Software is produced for which no specification was ever written down; the nearest thing to a specification is the programmer's own shifting intentions. Given the final product, there is the task of specifying it; this would be necessary for the purposes of documentation, maintenance, etc. All programmers know that it is extremely difficult to read a program text and discover what the program does; this is the problem of 'reverse engineering'. Difficult though the task is, it is actually quite well defined: to give an exhaustive characterization of the input/output relation defined by the program. Of course, unless the program is carefully designed to prevent it, many inputs will result in meaningless output, error messages or core dumps. The meaningful part of the program's functionality is restricted to those inputs for which such maverick behaviour does not occur, and part of the task of reverse engineering must be to identify this subset of the inputs. To the extent that this cannot be defined uniquely the program does not have a unique specification. In any case it does not have a unique specification, since there will always be alternative equally correct ways of describing what it does do, even granted that one has fixed on a particular set of input/output pairs as the ones for which we want to regard the program's behaviour as meaningful.

The reverse engineering problem can expressed as

> Given P, find an X such that P answers the question 'How can we do X?'.

We are, so to speak, looking for a converse to the question How? In computer science 'how?' is usually contrasted with 'what?': the specification says WHAT you want to achieve, the implementation says HOW to achieve it. However, WHAT is a rather weak word which can cover descriptions at many different levels.

You might see someone adding up a list of figures and ask them what they're doing. The answer 'I'm adding up this list of figures' might be sufficiently informative in some circumstances, but more likely the questioner will say, 'Yes, yes, I can see that, but why are you adding up the figures?', the required answer being something along the lines of 'I'm checking my bank balance' (though of course it might be 'Because teacher told me to'). The point is that the question *What?* often means *Why?*: one way of saying what one is doing is to say why one is doing it. A *what* that is totally uncontaminated by *why* could only be a description of the action as a *basic action* (Danto, 1965): not 'I'm checking my bank balance', not 'I'm adding up these figures', not even 'I'm writing down an "8" followed by a "7" . . .', or even 'I'm making a mark having such and such a shape and then to the right of that a mark having such and such another shape . . .', but only 'I've got my hand in such and such a position and moving it thus and so . . .'.

It is absolutely normal and commonplace to describe human actions in terms of their intended or actual effects (Anscombe, 1957). If the action is intentional then it will naturally be described in terms of 'action intended to have such and such an effect'; if unintentional, as 'action that in fact has such and such effects'. We make default assumptions about whether an action is intentional or not: 'He signed the cheque' is usually taken to be intentional, 'He knocked over the wine' as unintentional. But intentionality or otherwise is secondary to the fact of describing something in terms of its effects.

To see Y as an implementation of a specification X is to accept 'By doing Y' as an answer to the question 'How can we do X?', and equally to accept 'X' as an answer to the question 'What are they doing?' asked of someone who is seen to be doing Y.

In generalizing the specification/implementation distinction as we have begun to do, though, we are perhaps in danger of diluting the concept so much that nothing of value remains. At this point it is important to take stock of precisely what relationships we are prepared to countenance under the rubric specification/implementation.

In the first place, the specification of a system describes it from the outside: it as it were envisages the system as a kind of black box which can be observed to interact with its environment in various ways without giving any clue as to the internal mechanism responsible for those interactions. The implementation, on the other hand, consists precisely of the details of that mechanism. The implementational hierarchy discussed earlier in this section can be envisaged as follows: when we open up the black box, we do not immediately see all the details of the mechanism at once; what we see is a number of smaller black boxes connected to each other in various ways. If we know the function of each of the smaller black boxes and understand how these functions interact as a result of their visible interconnections, then we have at least a partial understanding of the mechanism of the big black box. But for a fuller understanding, we have to penetrate each of the smaller black boxes; and in a complex system, the number of levels of black boxes nested within other black boxes may be very large.

The black box picture suggests a second important relationship that is involved in the specification/implementation relation, already adumbrated in our talk of effect, which inevitably brings in the complementary notion of cause. Put crudely, it is that the specification is concerned with *effects*, the implementation with *causes*. We can think of a specification as describing the effects that the system to be built will manifest; and the successful implementation as a mechanism which causes exactly those effects.

There are at least two different notions of cause which might work here. Take the case of a program that is proved to meet a certain formal specification (one of our insertion sort programs would do as an example here). In what sense can we say that the program causes the behaviour described in the specification? One answer is that on a properly configured computer, running the program physically causes the generation of input/output pairs from amongst those given by the specification. As we saw above, though, this is not what is proved when one mathematically proves that the program meets its specification. Rather one proves that a certain formal relation holds between them that abstracts from the details of the actual physical computation and all the low-level systems that support it: in so far as we are still talking about causality here, it is more akin to Aristotle's notion of formal cause than to his notion of efficient cause. It is a nice point whether the formal relation is an abstract model of the physical computation or, as Fetzer would have it, the latter is a causal (i.e., efficient causal) model of the former.

On this point depends the view that we must take of the essential relationship between specification and implementation. Should we take the view that computation is essentially a physical process, and that the mathematical account of it is an abstraction, convenient for some purposes, on a par with the mathematical account of planetary motion, fluid flow, or business cycles? Or should we on the contrary take the view that computation is essentially mathematical in character and that the physical adjuncts of computation are only there in order to allow us as physical beings to grasp what is going on?

In support of the latter view, one might offer the thought that any physical implementation is inevitably incomplete with respect to an abstract specification. For example, one might specify an algorithm for finding the quotient and remainder when one of an arbitrary pair of non-negative integers is divided by the other; but any implementation of this is liable to fall foul of the fact that an actual physical computer is limited in the size of the integers it can represent, and hence its actual input/output behaviour will only amount to a vanishingly small fragment of the infinite range that is specified and which the abstract algorithm is adequate to handle in full. It is the same thought that in the theory of computation we regard our computational devices as having a power equivalent to that of a Turing machine rather than of a finite-state automaton, although given the actual physical limitations, the latter is strictly speaking the more nearly correct assumption.

In support of the alternative view, we may note that physicality is not a merely incidental feature of us and our computing machines: it is essential to our very nature. No computation is ever of the slightest use to us, or can even be said to exist for us at all, except in so far as it is realized physically, whether this be in the electronic circuitry of a computer, in pencil marks on paper, or in the neuronal activity of an individual's brain. Moreover, even the specifications of many software systems make essential reference to the physical: the specification of a graphical interface, for example, might refer to colours in the screen display. The whole point of such a specification is lost if the colours are replaced by abstract place-holders and the specification regarded as specifying a pure mathematical function—even though this latter view is in principle entirely possible.

What I am concerned to bring out here is the tension between what I might call the 'view from reality' and the 'view from abstraction'. Abstraction is a wonderful and indeed quite extraordinary faculty of the human brain: that we are able to mediate our dealings with the physical world by way of ideas is responsible for the unique position in which we find ourselves in relation to the rest of nature. At one level, though, our abstractions can all be described in physical terms as patterns in our brains, and yet so to describe them is precisely to miss the distinctive feature of them which is—their abstractness. It is necessary that they be realized physically since the world provides no other way of realizing them, but how they are realized is immaterial to their essential nature.

A correct view of the matter would seem to be something like this: a physical system S may be described at many different levels of abstraction. If D is a description of S at a certain level of abstraction then S may be regarded as a full implementation of D, and D as a specification of S. If D' is a description of S at a lower level of abstraction than D, then of course D' can still be regarded as a specification of S, but it can also be regarded as a partial implementation (or abstract implementation) of D, which in turn can be regarded as specifying D' as well as S.

Here we are assuming that D and D' do correctly describe S. More realistically we may be faced with an S, D, and D' for which we do not know for sure whether the correct relations hold. In that case there are several possibilities. Since D and D' are both descriptions, there is the possibility (depending on the form of language in which the descriptions are couched) that we can prove mathematically that for any physical system S, if D' correctly describes S then so does D. This is to prove that D' is a correct partial implementation of D. Of course it says nothing directly about any actual physical system S, and no result whose proof is purely mathematical can be expected to do so (this is the Fetzer point).

Alternatively, when a programmer says 'My program seems to work but I don't understand why it does', he is saying in effect that the physical system S which consists of the up-and-running version of his program is apparently correctly described by the specification D he is working to, but he is unaware of any intermediate description D' which could simultaneously serve as a correct partial implementation of D and a specification of S.

Finally, one might be confronted with a physical system S—as when one has on disc the compiled version of someone's program but not its source code, and no documentation either—for which one does not know any D which correctly describes it. The task of finding such a D is inevitably an empirical exercise—reverse engineering again (or 'decompilation').

2. A wider view

Apart from a brief excursus in which we considered ways of describing what someone is doing when they are adding up a column of figures, our discussion so far has concentrated solely on the process of software development. There are a number of ways in which we can naturally generalize the ideas we have expounded into adjacent fields. Consider for a start two ways in which computational concerns are thought to have relevance for wider scientific or technological purposes. On the one hand there is the problem of computational simulation of what are not, on the face of it, intrinsically computational phenomena; on the other there is the problem of using the concepts and methods of computer science in the description of such phenomena, to describe them *as if* they were in some sense computational in nature themselves. To both of these classes of problems the notions of specification and implementation are of relevance.

Where the non-computational domain consists of human mental phenomena, the former problem (computational simulation) is a central concern of Artificial Intelligence; the latter problem is likewise central to Cognitive Science, if by that title one wishes to understand the systematic investigation of human cognition using the conceptual tools afforded by the existence of the electronic computer.

In the computational domain, the objects of study—specifications, algorithms, programs, etc—are without exception artefactual. In the most highly disciplined programming, in which the specification is made explicit before an implementation is produced, there is an intentional act of specification which directly leads to the no less intentional act of implementation. Less rigorous methods of software development can better be described in terms of an emerging specification, which is perhaps never made explicit but only exists as a potential *post hoc* rationalization of the final product in relation to the demands that led to its production. A third possibility, which does not seem to occur in the computational sphere, but which will become increasingly prominent as we extend our investigations more widely, is that *neither* the specification nor the implementation is the product of an intentional act: rather, an object that has come into existence by whatever means may prove to be describable as if it were the implementation of some specification, which we may then call, to use a term introduced by Partridge (1986), a *de facto* specification.

If this seems a somewhat forced extension of our notion of specification, we need only consider this: to be able to describe an object X as an implementation of some *de facto* specification Y is already a step on the road to simulating X: for the specification Y can just as well be treated as representing an intention. And to know what criteria one has to meet in order successfully to simulate X is itself an important precondition for properly understanding X. In effect we are saying that the word 'implementation' displays 'process/product ambiguity', and in common with some other such terms there is the possibility of usefully applying it to objects which display all the characteristics implied by the 'product' sense of the term but without actually having arisen by the process denoted by the 'process' sense (as, for example, we can talk about the *measurements* of an object which has never, in fact, been measured).

The notion of *de facto* specification brings with it an interesting twist: for in this case the correctness relation is reversed. Here the implementation is a given, and we might put up for consideration a variety of different possible *de facto* specifications; the question then arises which of these specifications correctly describe what the implementation does. So we must speak of the correctness of a putative *de facto* specification relative to an implementation rather than the other way around.

A system can be regarded as analogous to a software system in so far as it can be regarded as a mechanism which meets some functional specification. There is, I suppose, a vacuous sense in which this is true of any physical system (I mean a system in a particular instantaneous state). Let I be the set of all possible ways in which the world outside the system could affect it ('inputs'), and let O be the set of all possible ways in which the system could affect the world outside it ('outputs'). Now, let $S \in I \times O$ be the set of input/output pairs that can occur for the system in the given state. Then we could say that the system meets the specification: Given input i, produce an output o such that $(i,o) \in S$.

A significant application of software engineering concepts outside the domain of software engineering should set some limits to how those concepts are to be interpreted in the wider domain. Some criterion is required for determining whether a description of how a system behaves can properly be described as a *de facto* specification of that system. Such criteria are not always easy to come by; we shall examine some important special cases in due course. In a general way, though, one conclusion which is suggested by the earlier discussion is that in order to count as an implementation of a given specification, a system should, in an appropriate environment, be able ultimately to cause the behaviour specified.

In order to test the viability of these ideas we shall embark on a series of case studies, in which we examine the applicability of the notions of specification and implementation in various *prima facie* non-computational fields, culminating in the field of most interest to cognitive science, the mind itself. Before embarking on the case studies, though, we first take a look at some related work in which, in effect, computational concepts are applied outside the field of computer science proper.

We begin with David Marr's celebrated trinity of levels (Marr, 1982). Marr was concerned to define the idea of a level of explanation for a complex system. He posited just three of them, namely

1. The *computational* level, at which the system is explained in terms of what it does, i.e., what function it computes, or its input/output behaviour.

2. The *algorithmic* level, at which a system is explained in terms of the computational procedures or algorithms by which it does what it does.

3. The *physical* or *implementational* level, at which a system is explained in terms of the physical mechanisms by which it does what it does.

In our terms, the computational level provides a high-level specification of the system. This will be *de facto* if our concern is with explaining an already given system, *ante hoc* if we are concerned with actually building the system. The algorithmic level provides one kind of implementation of the high-level specification; but itself serves as a specification in relation to the physical level. (This is the ambiguity in the notion of implementation which we noted above.)

Our earlier considerations would suggest that it is an oversimplification to posit just three levels in this way: the top two levels, in particular, grade into one another through a series of refinements—we illustrated this, crudely, with our sorting algorithms above. The first statement of the insertion-sort algorithm was partly algorithmic and partly computational, in as much as no algorithm was provided for the insertion component, only a specification. Again, between the 'pure' algorithmic level and the physical level we can interpose a sequence of intermediate steps, including the encoding of the algorithm as a program, the compilation of the program to machine code, the interpretation of the machine code as microcode, the execution of the microcode. As McClamrock (1991) has noted, any one of these stages can be regarded as representing the algorithmic level; from there we can look either upwards to the next higher-level stage—which we now regard as representing the computational level—or downwards to the next lower-level stage, representing the physical, or implementational, level. In McClamrock's words,

> The number of actual algorithmic levels of organization in any given information-processing system . . . is an entirely empirical

matter about that particular system . . .. But for each of those levels of organization . . ., there are three *perspectives* that we can take towards it—or if you prefer, three general kinds of questions that we can pose about it . . .: questions about that structure itself; questions about the functional, context-dependent properties of the parts and relations in that structure and their contribution to the functioning of the system as a whole; and questions about the implementation of the primitive parts of that algorithmic structure (McClamrock 1991, pp. 192–3).

Taking our earlier identification of the higher-level *What* as a kind of *Why*, we can correlate these three perspectives with the questions *Why?—What?—How?* The cleanness of the separation between these three types of questions will vary according to the design of the system one is looking at. In computing it is generally felt to be desirable to effect as clean a separation as possible, so that at each level the lower-level implementational details are effectively hidden—that, after all, is the whole point of high-level programming languages—and moreover the higher-level functionality subserved by that level likewise does not intrude.

I think McClamrock has provided a satisfactory solution to the question why it was natural for Marr to define just three levels rather than any other number; this notwithstanding attempts that have been made to interpose further levels in the Marr hierarchy (e.g., Peacocke, 1986). Such attempts would seem to take more seriously than is really warranted the supposition that Marr's levels are absolute rather than perspectival. Churchland and Sejnowski (1989) find flaws in both the tripartite character of Marr's conception and the notion of independence between the levels. Regarding the former, the perspectival interpretation seems an adequate response; as for the latter, the point is well taken, but is surely not fatal to Marr's conception—rather it brings to cognitive science the same point that Swartout and Balzer made about the inevitable intertwining of specification and implementation. The fact that the separation between the levels is not sharp does not invalidate the notion of levels altogether.

Another no less celebrated trinity is that of Dennett (1978). Dennett identifies three *stances* that we can take towards explaining or predicting the behaviour of a complex system; they are as follows:

1. The *physical* stance, which invokes the physical constitution of a system, and the physical nature of the impingements upon it, and uses the laws of physics to predict how the system will behave;

2. The *design* stance, which assumes that the system has a certain design, and predicts that it will behave as it is designed to behave under various circumstances;

3. The *intentional* stance, which treats the system as a rational agent, and predicts its behaviour from the beliefs and desires that it ought to have, given its circumstances.

As with Marr's levels, attempts have been made to elaborate Dennett's scheme by the inclusion of further stances (e.g., the ascriptional stance of Narayanan, 1990).

It is tempting to try to correlate Dennett's stances with Marr's levels; the correlation seems to start off well, with the physical level corresponding to the physical stance. The algorithmic level likewise corresponds with the design stance, in that an algorithm can be thought of as a design—although as soon as we remember that we can talk of higher or lower levels of design, and that the higher levels grade into the lower levels through a series of refinement steps, we realise that things are a little more complicated. It is at the top level that the two systems do not seem to match so well. To describe a system at Marr's computational level is, essentially, to describe its functionality; it is not to ascribe to it beliefs and desires. If anything, it is to ascribe beliefs and desires to the designer of the system, but even this cannot literally apply in the case of systems which arose through processes other than being deliberately designed.

3. Case study 1: Group action

Anscombe (1957) introduced the idea of an action's being intentional or not 'under a description'. Davidson (1971) gives as an example: I switch on the light and thereby alert a prowler. It is a single action, and it is an intentional action on my part; but it is only intentional under the description 'switching on the light' and not under the description 'alerting the prowler'. That way Anscombe is able to draw a distinction between acting intentionally and acting with a certain intention: in doing what I did when I alerted the prowler I was acting intentionally, but it was not the intention of my action *to* alert the prowler, only to switch on the light.

Now although Anscombe's idea specifically subserves her ulterior purpose of analysing intention, it finds ready application outside the realm of the intentional too. As we have seen, a good way of thinking about specifications and implementations is in terms of a hierarchy of correct descriptions of what a computer system does. This is in many ways comparable to the sort of hierarchy of descriptions that Anscombe constructs for human actions. She has an example in which a man's action is describable as moving his arm up and down, pumping, replenishing the water supply, poisoning the inhabitants of the house, and bringing about the revolution. Each term of this series can be regarded as describing an implementation of the next one along, which in turn could be regarded as a specification, whether *de facto*, *post hoc*, or *ante hoc*, of each of its predecessors.

Now a point which is absolutely crucial for a correct understanding of the relationships involved here is that in describing an action in a particular way we are almost always going beyond the local physical phenomena to include features of the environment within which those phenomena occur. In Anscombe's example, the man's moving his arm up and down only *is* pumping because it takes place in a context in which the man is holding the handle of a working pump. And the pumping is only replenishing the water supply of the house because the pump is connected to the house's plumbing arrangements in the right way. And replenishing the water supply is only poisoning the inhabitants because the water is poisoned and the inhabitants are drinking it. And poisoning the inhabitants is only bringing about the revolution because the inhabitants are key figures on whose elimination the success of the revolution depends.

Anscombe's hierarchy illustrates well the threefold scheme *Why?—What?—How?* by which we encapsulated McClamrock's perspectival reinterpretation of Marr's three levels. Suppose we see the man in Anscombe's example and ask 'What is he doing?' As answer, he could give any of the descriptions we have considered—moving his arm up and down, pumping, replenishing the water supply, and so on. Whichever answer he gives, we can go on to ask two further questions, namely 'Why is he doing that?' and 'How is he doing it?'. The 'why' question looks further along the series towards the more inclusive description, e.g., he's moving his arm up and down in order to pump, and pumping in order to replenish the water supply, which he is doing in order to poison the inhabitants, and so on. The 'how' question looks in the opposite direction: he's bringing about the revolution by poisoning the inhabitants, which he is doing by replenishing the water supply, which he is doing by pumping, and so on.

In terms of human action, the series must come to an end eventually, in either direction: one has ends which are desired for their own sake, not as a means to anything else (so the question 'why?' is inappropriate); and there are actions (so-called *basic actions*) which one does not do by doing anything else, one just does them. On the other hand, if one is prepared to go beyond descriptions of human actions *qua* actions, and consider, at the 'lower' end of the scale, the physiological processes involved in bodily movements, and at the 'higher' end, the social interactions of which individual human actions can form a part, we see that the series becomes more open-ended in nature. Thus, while under normal conditions we can't reasonably ask someone 'How did you raise your arm?' (the only appropriate answer is 'I just did'), we *can* ask, a propos of the body itself, considered as a mechanism, 'By what physiological processes is the arm-raising accomplished?', the answer being perhaps given in terms of a signal sent out from the motor cortex of the brain giving rise to contraction of a certain muscle.

Likewise, our pumping man may be merely the agent of some revolutionary organization, which may be considered in some sense to make decisions, carry out actions, and generally to *bear responsibility* in a way that goes beyond the activities of any of its constituent individuals (who, from this perspective, may be mere 'cogs in a machine'). Our man may in fact be unaware that in replenishing the water supply he is poisoning the inhabitants of the house and thereby bringing about the revolution; but these further ends may still be the real purposes of his action, not from his own individual standpoint but from the point of view of the organization to which he owes allegiance. And indeed it could be that the organization is so compartmentalized that no one individual is in possession of the information that this man's pumping is to be instrumental in bringing about the revolution, even though precisely this is a consequence of all the information possessed by all the members of the organization.

These leads us naturally to the main theme of this section: Group Action. We here consider groups of people, such as committees, performing tasks that are paradigmatically done by individuals. Aaron Sloman has suggested to me that this should be regarded as a form of implementation; and indeed we seem here to be on the borderline between artefacts and natural objects.

The issue here is whether a committee really makes a decision or whether it merely simulates the decision-making process that we find in individual humans. One reason why this is important is that it has some bearing on the individual case: for example, someone might claim that when an individual human decides something, there is actually a 'committee' of homunculi in his brain which makes the decision collectively. For this to work, it is important to show how a committee can make a decision as a group without any member of the committee making it as an individual. Suppose that the committee members put forward a number of suggestions, whose relative merits they discuss, and then they take a vote. Finally the edict is pronounced: the committee has decided not to raise the subscription this year. No individual member of the committee can claim to have decided that, not even the ones who voted for it; what they can all claim is that they took part in the decision-making process. But this means merely that they participated in the mechanism by which the abstract notion of deciding was implemented in this particular case.

We can say that the action of deciding, considered as a specification, can be implemented in various ways. One way is by means of a committee. Another way is by tossing a coin. Yet another way is by that distinctive type of individual human action to which we paradigmatically apply the word 'deciding'. We can agree to this whether or not we accept the idea that in the individual the action is implemented by means of an internal committee. As we have emphasised above, it is a distinctive feature of the notions of specification and implementation that one and the same specification can be implemented in many radically different ways.

Where a committee is set up with a constitution that explicitly regulates the kinds of decision-making processes that are to be allowed to it, we may think of the committee as an artefact, and the process of setting it up an implementation in the process sense. But sometimes committees arise in an informal way when groups of concerned individuals come together and collectively make decisions without ever having established any agreed mechanisms for doing so. An *ad hoc* committee of this kind is much less like an artefact, and while we may still wish to regard it as an implementation, in the 'product' sense, of the abstract specification of deciding, it becomes much less plausible to say that it is an implementation in the 'process' sense.

An obvious objection here is that if no individuals ever made decisions, then no committee could either; that collective decision is dependent on the existence of individual decisions. Thus in our subscription example, while it is true that no individual decided not to raise the subscription (although a majority of them voted for this), it is *not* true that no individual made a decision. Each individual decided how to vote (or abstain), each individual at some point decided, at least implicitly, that they would abide by the collectively agreed decision-making process, and so on. If these individual decisions are implemented by committees of homunculi, then the question only gets pushed back further to the individual homuncular decision-making processes. However, as Dennett

127

points out, the trick is to implement each homunculus in terms of *less clever* homunculi, until 'they have been reduced to functionaries "who can be replaced by a machine" ' (Dennett, 1978, Ch. 5).

These considerations lead us to a rejection of essentialism with regard to processes such as decision-making. Naively, one supposes that what makes a process one of *deciding* is that it partakes in some mysterious way of a special quality that makes it a decision rather than anything else—as it were a *virtus constitutiva* which is possessed by the human soul but not by any mere mechanism. We now see that what makes a process one of deciding is rather that it meets a certain specification: in particular, it must have the right effect on the subsequent actual or potential behaviour of the decision-maker. This means that, as we have noted, decision-making can be implemented in many different ways, in decision-makers of many different kinds. Nothing is *merely* a decision-maker; rather a system that makes decisions plays host to a virtual 'decider' that implements the specification of decision-making.

4. Case study 2: Morphogenesis

The genetic code has often been likened to a programming language, and an individual genome to a program written in that language. Of course this is only a metaphor if by 'program' we understand something consciously and deliberately designed by an individual. The designer of genomes is rather the Blind Watchmaker of Dawkins (1986), which is to say that it is a virtual designer implemented in the medium of natural selection. However, we have already seen that just as important to the notion of a program as a deliberately engineered artefact is the notion of a program as the implementation of a specification. If, then, a genome is to be regarded in this light as a program, what is its specification?

We can, perhaps, think of a genome as implementing a specification of the form 'creature optimally adapted to such-and-such a way of life in such-and-such an environment'; the organism itself is the result of 'executing' the genome in a particular environment. More exactly, taking our cue from Dawkins' concept of the extended phenotype (Dawkins, 1982), we can say that an environment, together with all the organisms it contains, is the result of executing the genomes of all those organisms in that environment. The circularity here is only perfect in the case of a completely stable, unevolving environment that has no beginning in time. In reality, environments are never perfectly stable, and we should rather say that the environment at time t is the result of the genomes' being executed in the environment at times $t-\delta$ (where δ varies according to the individual organism)—thus discharging the circularity, and opening a 'loophole' for natural selection to get to work.

We earlier made the point that in general a system will constitute an implementation of a specification only in the context of some environment in which it is, or can be, embedded. The specification may itself extend to a description of the effects that the system has on its environment (this feature is already present in the case of quite simple computer programs whose purpose is to direct the operation of various peripheral devices—which of course form part of the environment in which the program is running). The present case study illustrates this point well. To borrow an example from Dawkins, the *de facto* specification that is met by the genome of a beaver includes far-reaching effects on the environment wrought by the beaver's habit of constructing dams which can affect the flow of the river, and with it its ecology, for a considerable distance both upstream and downstream. And the essential point made by Dawkins is that these 'environmental' elements of the *de facto* specification also play a part in defining the overall selection pressures on the genome and hence are of relevance to its further evolution.

Since an organism is a complex system with many interlocking subsystems, we can readily view it (or its genome) as implementing many different partial specifications. And once again we see that a given specification can be implemented in many different ways. Thus the specification 'creature capable of flying through the air' is implemented quite differently by insects, pterosaurs, birds, and bats; the differences in the implementations can to some extent be attributed to the fact that the specification has to be met alongside a whole host of additional specifications or partial implementations (for example, internal *v.* external skeleton, endothermy *v.* exothermy, ovipary *v.* vivipary). The phenomenon of convergent evolution (as for example in the often-cited streamlining of sharks, dolphins, and ichthyosaurs) shows conversely that even though a specification can be met in many different ways, there may be comparatively few viable high-level designs for a given specification. Equally, certain well tried and tested 'programming tricks' may be preserved unaltered for many millions of years, witness the remarkably constant form of the haemoglobin molecule over a wide range of different animal phyla.

This last example suggests a further parallel between the biological and software engineering domains. As we noted above, there is in reality a gradation between the highest-level specification of a software system and its low-level physical description, with inter-mediate levels which can be simultaneously viewed as partial implementations of the higher levels and specifications of the lower. Biological organisms can be described in terms of exactly the same kind of hierarchical organization. The specification of the haemoglobin molecule would refer primarily to its oxygen-carry-ing capacity, including the precise circumstances under which it will take up an oxygen atom or release it. This specification would not form a part of a gross functional specification of the whole organism, which would rather refer to its locomotive, alimentary, and reproductive capacities, amongst others. To implement this higher level specification, though, one of the requirements is an efficient system for the distribution of raw materials and energy; one way of implementing this is by means of a bloodstream with certain specified capacities. The energetic aspect is implemented, in part, by specifying an oxygen-transportation system, in the implementation of which haemoglobin plays a key role. It may not be the uniquely best way of doing it, but its persistence through-out otherwise far-reaching evolutionary changes suggests that it is at least a clear local optimum.

One difficulty with all this is once again the familiar one of determining what the specification is in a given case. If we are to justify our claim that genomes are like programs by appeal to the consideration that they, like programs, can be viewed as imple-mentations of specifications, then we had better have a robust notion of what specifications a genome implements; otherwise the conception lapses into vacuity. For this reason, the question which so often plagues biologists—'what is the adaptive function of this feature of this organism?'—is of paramount importance here. For in seeking the evolutionary *raison d'être* of such-and-such an anatomical, physiological, or behavioural feature, one is, precisely, looking for a specification, in the form given above, that is imple-mented by the relevant part of the creature's genome. Some biolo-gists hold that not all features of an organism are there because they have conferred a reproductive advantage on the organism's ancestors; but rather that some just 'happen' to have arisen, and being neither advantageous nor disadvantageous have persisted for lack of any mutation away from them. Such 'neutral' features—or rather the portions of the genome which they express—cannot so easily be regarded as programs, precisely because their *de facto* effects are uncoupled from the mechanism of natural selection which could most naturally confer upon them the status of speci-fications.

The appropriateness of applying the language of software engineering to biology is enhanced by the advent of biology's own engineering discipline, genetic engineering. It is entirely natural to speak of a genetic engineer *programming* a bacterium to produce human insulin, say, with the genetic code as the programming language and DNA the hardware in which it is implemented. It does not seem that we can any longer draw a hard and fast distinction between human purposes on the one hand and the 'virtual purposes' that we find in nature on the other. Mayr (1988) distinguishes between *teleonomic* processes, which 'owe [their] goal-directedness to the operation of a program', where a program is defined to consist of 'coded or prearranged information that controls a process (or behaviour) leading it towards a given end', and *teleological* processes, which are guided towards their goal by purposive forces immanent in the world. He inclines to the view that there is no genuine teleology in the world, by which I take it he means that all apparently teleological processes can in fact be explained as teleonomic ones. (This is analogous to Dennett's view that even where the intentional stance is appropriate, explanation of behaviour could in principle be given in terms of the design stance, and ultimately the physical stance—this is reductionism of a kind, but not the simple-minded kind of reductionism that insists that beliefs, intentions, etc, do not really exist at all; they exist, all right, but as *implementations* in a medium that could in principle be described in terms belonging to a lower level of description.)

One of the most beautiful analogies between genomes and programs is the one between natural viruses and computer viruses. All existing computer viruses, as far as I know, have been deliberately contrived as such by malevolent or mischievous programmers. Perhaps the final vindication of the view that genomes and programs are fundamentally similar would be if a computer virus were to arise naturally out of a chance collocation of 'garbage' in the memory of some computer, with all the powers of dispersal possessed by the artificial kind. Such a virus would be sinister indeed, and all the more difficult to control, since the principles of its construction would doubtless be quite alien to us when compared with those that have been created by humans.

5. Case study 3: The Mind

This section could well have been included as a part of the previous one, for the mind too is a feature of the human organism and thus can be investigated from an evolutionary standpoint. In particular, however little we may understand about the details of the process, it it is hard to avoid the conclusion that the possession of a mind (whatever this ultimately amounts to) is coded for in the human genome by virtue of the instructions for building a brain. We here set on one side the long-running controversy over just what properties of the mind are so encoded, and to what degree—it being obvious that *some* properties of the developed mind (for example the propensity to think in English rather than Russian) are not genotypic but rather arise from the interaction of genetically programmed faculties with the environment in which the individual finds itself.

The reason why the mind deserves a section on its own is that its relevance to our theme goes beyond the purely evolutionary perspective of the previous section. The brain is unique amongst the organs of the body in its resemblance to a computer. The many analogies and disanalogies are too well-known to bear repeating here; what is important for us is the perspective by which mental processes may be regarded as analogous to the execution of computer programs—or whole suites of such programs. Setting aside for the moment the question of how just this analogy really is, it raises for us the immediate question: if the mind is a program, what specification does it implement? On the view propounded above, it is only reasonable to regard the mind as a program to the extent that we can meaningfully answer this question.

The quest for a single overarching (and inevitably highly complicated) specification for a human mind would seem to be futile. A human being participates in an enormous range of different kinds of interaction with its environment; a functional specification of the mind of that human would require a complete characterization of the possible inputs to it—and this would mean not just categorizing the physical impingements of the environment on the human body, but more specifically deciding which of those impingements are to count as inputs to the mind, and in what form they should be represented; in addition, many internal bodily phenomena should doubtless also be classed as inputs to the mind. The problem of output is just as complex; and then beyond that we should require a comprehensive account of the relationship between possible inputs and possible outputs. Many of these questions will have answers that are highly indeterminate: and this opens up the possibility that there are many possible specifications which a given mind can be regarded as meeting (cf. Dennett, 1978, Ch.13).

It seems that the only way we can possibly make any headway in this enterprise is by looking for 'local' specifications which cover restricted portions of a human's mental functioning. Are there subsystems of the human mind which can be described, without doing violence to the complexity of the whole, as implementations meeting a given functional specification?

To some extent, it seems that there are. As a simple example, we can observe by introspection that there are many instances in which a stimulus is invariably followed by a particular kind of mental event. For instance, it is very hard for a literate English speaker, on being presented with the visual stimulus

$$\boxed{\text{BOOT}}$$

not to think of a boot, while at the same time most probably hearing in the mind's ear the sound sequence /bu:t/. The details of this reaction doubtless differ from person to person: 'thinking of a boot' will involve a network of associations involving visual, tactile or perhaps olfactory representations, and the details of this network will be peculiar to the individual concerned. But whatever is really going on when things appear to the mind's eye or ear, phenomena such as these have the hallmarks of a program which responds selectively to different inputs according to what we are inclined to describe as their 'meaning'. And the program is obviously not innate: the same stimulus BOOT, when presented to a literate German-speaker, will instead evoke the image of a *boat*, and the sound sequence /bo:t/.

For us, the important issue is whether the complex network of actions and reactions in the mind can be viewed as the workings of a program constructed in accordance with some specification. Of course, the specification must be merely implicit, most of the time; only the most formal parts of our education can be construed as an explicit *engineering* of our mental apparatus. But if we consider the way in which language is learnt, it does seem that the speech habits of the community into which an individual is born constitute an implicit specification to which the child's developing language tends to converge (never completely, not least because the community in question is ill-defined at the edges, and its speech-habits likewise). If, as Chomsky maintains, there is a universal grammar 'hard-wired' into the brain, then the difficult, structural part of the program is already largely in place at birth, and only requires exposure to the speech-habits of a particular community for adjusting the settings of various parameters.

The possible roles of grammatical theory can, perhaps, be clarified a little by the software engineering perspective we have advocated. For consider the spirit in which a formal grammar for a particular language is presented. On the one hand, its advocates might claim that the grammar reflects, at a certain level of description, the actual implementation of the language in the brain: that is, the processes abstractly described in the grammar directly reflect processes going on in our minds or brains when we use the language. On the other hand, more modestly (and perhaps more realistically), one could claim that the grammar presents only a functional specification of the language: it purports to define what sentences the language contains, perhaps associating them with meanings too, but lays no claim to an account of how the linguistic faculty is actually implemented in the brain. This is somewhat analogous to the controversy over the role that formal logic plays in both software engineering and artificial intelligence. For on the one hand, ambitious attempts have been made to use formal logic as an implementation tool, that is, to use it as the basis for programming languages (e.g., in logic programming) or program synthesis systems; on the other hand, there is the view that it is only suited to playing the role of a specification language, the actual implementation being conducted by altogether different means. My own inclination, in this case, as in the case of language and the brain, is towards the view of 'formal-system-as-specification-language' rather than 'formal-system-as-implementation-technology'.

Of course, language is only one part of our mental equipment, and it may be that if we look at other parts, the notion that our mental faculties are implementations of specifications may seem less appropriate. Still, we may recall here Marr's trinity of levels, which as we mentioned above can be thought of, following McClamrock, as enshrining the implementation/specification distinction in the context of the different perspectives we may adopt when attending to any particular level of description of a complex system. And we should remember that Marr's trinity was proposed in the first instance as a way of thinking about the problems of understanding *vision*—which for those of us lucky enough to be sighted constitutes a major part of our mental life.

6. Conclusions

In conclusion, we may sum up our findings as follows. The distinction between specification and implementation arises naturally in the context of computer programming as a way of providing a firm foundation for the notion of a program's being correct or otherwise. The distinction is not, however, an absolute one, but must be regarded as a relation between stages in the development of a program. Every specification is itself an implementation of a specification at a higher level (Swartout and Balzer 1983). A similar relation exists in the field of human action, in which a given action can be described variously in terms of its intended or actual effect at various removes (Anscombe 1957). In both these cases we can, at each level in an implementational hierarchy, look 'up' towards a higher-level description in terms of more global effects and purposes or 'down' towards a lower-level description in terms of local mechanisms: this gives us a three-fold division which may be identified, following McClamrock, with Marr's well-known trinity of levels.

The relationship between specification and implementation can be viewed as that between a description of a system as a 'black box' and a description which reveals what is inside the black box. Specifically, what is required is a description of the interior of the box *as a mechanism* with the power to produce the effects described by the specification. This led us to consider the role of causality in supporting a description of something as an implementation of a specification: in particular, we suggested that something can be regarded as an implementation of a given specification only in a context in which it is ultimately able to cause the behaviour specified. And we examined the objection to this that in the field of computer programming we can at least in some cases regard *every* stage as a pure mathematical abstraction, with no essential physicality at all.

We next considered the possibility of taking a broader view, already adumbrated, to some extent, by the comparison with Anscombe's hierarchy of levels of description of human action. We noted that both the terms 'specification' and 'implementation' displayed product/process ambiguity, which led us to consider to what extent these terms can be significantly applied outside the realm of designed artefacts. We adopted the view that likening a complex system to a computer program is justifiable only in so far as the system can be regarded as the implementation (whether artefactual or not) of some specification.

We illustrated the potential illumination afforded by this perspective by looking at three specific cases: group action, morphogenesis, and the human mind. A lot of open questions were left, which reflects, in part, the fact that there is much that we do not yet know about how such systems actually work, but also in part the fact that we are still groping for a settled terminology for the description of complex systems. It is implicit in the discussions above that the natural place for us to look for such terminology is the world of computing: only the most complex of human artefacts, it seems, can provide a model for the complexities of nature.

References

Anscombe, G. E. M. 1957. *Intention*. Oxford: Basil Blackwell.

Churchland P. S. and Sejnowski, T. J. 1989. 'Neural representation and neural computation', in L. Nadel, L. Cooper, P. Culicover and R. M. Harnish (eds), *Neural Connections, Mental Computations*. Cambridge, Mass.: MIT Press.

Danto, A. C. 1965. 'Basic Actions', *American Philosophical Quarterly*, **2**, 141–148.

Davidson, D. 1971. *Agency*, in R. Binkley *et al.* (eds), *Agent, Action, and Reason*. University of Toronto Press. Reprinted in D. Davidson, 1980, *Essays on Actions and Events*, Oxford: Clarendon Press.

Dawkins, R. 1982. *The Extended Phenotype*. W. H. Freeman and Co.

Dawkins, R. 1986. *The Blind Watchmaker*. Longman.

Dennett, D. 1978. *Brainstorms*. Montgomery, Vermont: Bradford Books.

Fetzer, J. H. 1988. 'Program verification: the very idea', *Communications of the ACM*, **31** (9), 1048–1063.

Marr, D. 1982, *Vision*. W. H. Freeman & Co.

Mayr, E. 1988. *Toward a New Philosophy of Biology*. Cambridge, Mass.: Harvard University Press.

McClamrock, R. 1991. 'Marr's three levels: A re-evaluation', *Minds and Machines*, **1**, 185–196.

Narayanan, A. 1990. *On Being a Machine. Volume 2: Philosophy of Artificial Intelligence*. Chichester: Ellis Horwood.

Partridge, D. 1986. *Artificial Intelligence: applications in the future of software engineering*. Chichester: Ellis Horwood.

Peacocke, C. 1986. 'Explanation in computational psychology: language, perception and level 1.5', *Mind and Language*, **1**(2), 101–123.

Swartout, W. and Balzer, R. 1983. 'On the inevitable intertwining of specification and implementation', *Communications of the ACM*, **25**(7), 438–440.

Wittgenstein and Connectionism: a Significant Complementarity?*

STEPHEN MILLS

I

Between the later views of Wittgenstein and those of connection-ism[1] on the subject of the mastery of language there is an impressively large number of similarities. The task of establishing this claim is carried out in the second section of this paper (with arguments in the fourth section lending further support).

Having established the claim, I raise the question of the significance, if any, of the fact that there are these similarities between the two positions. In the first part of the third section I argue that the fact is theoretically important. However this conclusion is swiftly joined by another, viz., that the account of the similarities makes evident that between the positions there is also a difference of clear theoretical importance.

Can these two conclusions be reconciled? Later in the third section it is argued that they can, in the proposal that the views of Wittgenstein and connectionism are complementary in a theoretically important way. Finally in this section I present an argument for accepting the proposal.

Objections to this proposal can be anticipated and several are examined in the fourth section. It is shown that none of those examined is successful and, indeed, in some cases, that a proper

*Earlier papers on the relationship between Wittgenstein's philosophy and connectionism were read in April 1989 in Galway, at the Irish Philosophical Society conference on Wittgenstein's philosophy, and in April 1991 at Middle East Technical University, Ankara, and the Philosophy of Science conference in Dubrovnik. I am grateful for comments made at those presentations. The present paper is a substantially revised version of the paper read in September 1992 at the RIP conference on Philosophy and the Cognitive Sciences in Birmingham. Again I am grateful for comments and, in making revisions, I found those by Colin Radford, Stephen Stich, and Andrew Woodfield especially useful.

[1] Styles of connectionist modelling and interpretations of connectionism vary considerably. In order to make my discussion manageable I will generally intend 'connectionism' to refer to the well known position developed by Paul Smolensky (1987, 1988, 1991).

understanding of the issues raised serves to reinforce the view that the two positions are significantly complementary. While it will be evident that I am sympathetic to both positions as outlined, it is beyond the scope of this paper to argue either in their support or in their defence.

II

When we use or understand language we are not operating a symbolic calculus according to exact rules. This negative thesis, that our mastery of language is not subserved by the operations of a symbolic calculus, besides being stated explicitly (Wittgenstein 1969, p. 25; 1958, § 81), is an important underlying theme of Wittgenstein's later philosophy. That it assumes special importance is not surprising since it expresses the rejection of a fundamental thesis of the *Tractatus*.

Similarities with connectionism are immediately evident.

First, rejection of the symbolic calculus theory of language mastery is explicit in and crucially important to Smolensky's interpretation. We display language mastery on account of operations of an intuitive processor and these numerical operations are wholly different from those of a symbolic calculus (Smolensky 1988).

Secondly, just as Wittgenstein's rejection of the symbolic calculus view assumes special importance in contrast with the rival theory of the *Tractatus*, so does Smolensky's rejection in contrast with the rival theory of the symbolic paradigm.

Thirdly, for Smolensky, the claim that the symbolic calculus theory is false is a contingent, empirical claim; likewise Wittgenstein's claim is not that the calculus theory could not be true but that it is not true, and he points to obvious facts in its support (1969, p. 25).

Finally, there is a more complex agreement. Wittgenstein, of course, does not deny that a person can be said to follow a linguistic rule in such senses as that there may be a hypothesis which satisfactorily explains his use of a word, or that there is a 'rule which he looks up when he uses signs', or that there is a rule 'which he gives us in reply if we ask him what his rule is' (1958, § 82); nor that 'in *normal* cases . . . the use of a word is clearly prescribed' in the sense that 'we . . . are in no doubt . . . what to say in this or that case' (1958, § 142, my emphasis). However, the conjunction of these points with his rejection of the symbolic calculus theory entails that when we are following linguistic rules, in these ordinary senses, we are not doing so in virtue of operating a symbolic calculus. Smolensky also does not deny that we follow rules, linguistic or otherwise. Where a symbolic hypothesis successfully accounts for a person's use of a word we have a case of a system which appears to be operating with 'hard' rules but whose processing in fact is fundamentally 'soft'. And in the extreme case where a person consciously and explicitly follows a linguistic rule, while it will be 'natural' to model the processing involved symbolically, this processing in fact is non-symbolic and at best the model is a fairly accurate approximation (Smolensky 1988).[2]

Among Wittgenstein's reasons for rejecting the calculus view the most pertinent is that the ordinary words we use and understand lack exact definitions (1969, p. 25; 1958, § 66ff). First, for a given word, there is no exact definition in terms of what is common to the uses of the word, for there is no such common feature or set of features. The various uses of a word are unified, not by something they have in common, but by 'a complicated network of similarities overlapping and criss-crossing', similarities which are analogous to 'the various resemblances between members of a family' (1958, §§ 66, 67). Secondly, for a given word, there is no exact definition of the different kind which reflection on the family resemblances point may suggest, viz., a definition in terms of the logical sum of the word's different uses. One may legislatively define a word in this way, of course, but the resulting usage will not be that which we have mastered: the definition will have given the usage boundaries whereas the one which we have mastered has no boundaries. These points are more loosely expressed in Wittgenstein's remark that

> there are words of which one might say: They are used in a thousand different ways which gradually merge into one another. No wonder that we can't tabulate strict rules for their use. (1969, p. 28)

Wittgenstein's account of word usage has obvious similarities with Smolensky's account of representations within connectionist networks (1987, 1991). Smolensky develops his account with reference to an example, the connectionist representation of 'coffee'. He points out that if one takes the connectionist representation of 'cup with coffee' and subtracts from it the connectionist representation of 'cup without coffee', the result is not, as one might expect, the connectionist representation of 'coffee'. Rather the result is *a* connectionist representation of 'coffee' internal to which

---

[2] Mills (1990) discusses in detail the senses in which Smolensky is and is not eliminativist about symbolic processing; Mills (1992) challenges the non-eliminativist elements in his interpretation.

are references to the context in which coffee is in a cup. How one is to understand the notion of *the* connectionist representation of 'coffee' is then explained:

> The point is that the representation of 'coffee' that we get out of the construction starting with 'cup with coffee' leads to a different representation of 'coffee' than we get out of other constructions that have equivalent status *a priori* [e.g. 'can with coffee', 'tree with coffee']. This means that if you want to talk about the connectionist representation of 'coffee' in this distributed scheme, you have to talk about a *family of distributed activity patterns*. What knits together all these particular representations is nothing other than a *family resemblance* (1987, p. 148).

Apart from their actual use of the same term, 'family resemblance', the most obvious similarities between the two accounts concern the claims which this term is used to articulate.

First, employing Smolensky's example for both accounts, the claims, in their negative aspect, are, respectively, that the various uses of the word 'coffee' are not unified by features common to all and that the same is true of the various connectionist representations of 'coffee'. One general expression of this similarity would be that just as for Wittgenstein there literally are no such things as classical concepts or word meanings so for Smolensky there literally are no such things as classical symbols.

Secondly, and now positively, each claim asserts, of its respective field, that the principle of unification is one of overlapping and criss-crossing similarities.

There are also similarities which do not turn upon the family resemblances claims.

First, there is a similar reaction to non-standard calculus theories. As noted, Wittgenstein rejects not only theories which presuppose essentialist-type definitions of words but also theories which rely upon more complex, non-standard definitions. His reason is that for all their complexity—and what we might call apparent fuzziness—such formalisms place precise limits on word usage when, in fact, none exist. Smolensky also explicitly distinguishes these formalisms from his own position and expresses his opposition as follows:

> In [these formalisms] . . . softness is defined to be degrees of hardness. One takes the ontology of the problem that comes out of the hard approach, and one affixes numbers to all the elements of this ontology rather than reconceptualizing the ontology that intrinsically reflects the softness in the system (1987, p. 139).

The 'softness in the system' to which Smolensky refers is analogous to the lack of boundaries in word usage which Wittgenstein describes so that the positions are similar both in their rejections of the formalisms and their reasons for doing so.

Two further similarities emerge if one considers two ways in which, according to Wittgenstein, the lack of precise limits in a word's usage can be displayed. One of these is where usage is unproblematically extended to a genuinely new kind of case on the basis of similarities to one or more existing kinds. Here the resemblance is to the much stressed capacity of connectionist systems to recognize examples of a type which differ significantly from those employed in the training set. Lack of precise limits in a word's usage is also displayed in the fact that '[t]he more abnormal the case, the more doubtful it becomes what we are to say' (1958, § 142). Arguably this gradual increase in uncertainty is resembled by the way in which, in connectionist networks, there is gradual deviation from the desired output vector as examples become increasingly abnormal relative to the training set.

A final similarity between Wittgenstein's account of a word's usage and Smolensky's of representations concerns their respective treatment of the role of context. As noted earlier, on Smolensky's view, for any of the various representations of 'coffee' the context in which 'coffee' occurs is represented by internal features of the representation. One cannot then individuate a given representation of 'coffee' without making reference to the context in which the coffee occurs. Precisely the same is true for any of the various uses of a word on Wittgenstein's account. Since a given use is legitimate only within a certain kind of context one cannot individuate that use without referring to kinds of contextual features.

The last set of similarities to be itemized in this section may be introduced by noting that Wittgenstein's rejection of definitional accounts of word meaning inevitably raises the question of how language mastery is possible. Wittgenstein's answer is that we learn language, initially by drilling and training, then, once rudimentary understanding has developed, by teaching which employs a variety of intra-linguistic methods. Among the latter, explanations by means of examples and with reference to contexts are paramount. As will be familiar, the terms 'training' and 'learning' feature prominently in the connectionist literature: *learning* algorithms are employed for *training* up networks. However, as with 'family resemblance', one need not rely on mere usage of the same words to point out evident similarities with the Wittgensteinian position. First, while applying 'learning' and 'training' to networks doubtless involves new uses of the words, it is not difficult to think of existing uses which these new ones resemble. Secondly, since a set of examples is used in training up networks and, in the type of case discussed by Smolensky, specification of context features essentially, there are parallels here also with Wittgenstein's account.

III

The preceding comparison of the views of Wittgenstein and connectionism on the topic of linguistic mastery reveals an impressive number of similarities. Is this fact of theoretical importance? In this subsection I will argue that it is.

The first reason for holding that the fact is theoretically important is that the similarities are between theoretically important elements of the two positions. It cannot be doubted that the elements are theoretically important for they are fundamental or central to the accounts. Thus, to take a pair of negative elements, the rejection of the symbolic calculus theory of language mastery could hardly be more fundamental to either position: in Wittgenstein's case it marks a decisive break with what is foundational to his earlier position; in Smolensky's case it marks an equally decisive break with classical cognitivism. On the positive side, commitment to a full-blooded learning theory in which training based on examples plays an essential role is a central element of both accounts. Now if the similarities had held between evidently trivial or accidental elements then, whatever their number, there would be no reason to regard the fact of their existence as theoretically important. However, that theoretically important aspects are involved in all of many cases is a substantial reason for holding that the fact of the similarities is theoretically important.

A second reason is that between aspects which have been shown to be similar there are second order structural similarities which are of theoretical importance. By 'structural similarities' I mean similarities of either logical or functional role between paired features. Thus an important reason for Wittgenstein's rejection of the symbolic calculus view is that a word's various uses are unified only by family resemblances, while an important reason for Smolensky's rejection of the symbolic calculus view of classical cognitivism is that the various connectionist representations of, say, 'coffee' are united only by family resemblances. And in both accounts the notion of training and the reliance upon examples play similar functional roles in the respective learning theories.

A third reason can be gleaned from considering one aspect of certain assimilations against which there is a familiar Wittgensteinian move. The move is to caution against assimilations which are achieved at the price of blindness to what is really important about the assimilated phenomena, (certain of) their differences (1958, §§ 13–14). One aspect of such assimilations is that typically the purported similarity itself is in some way objectionable, e.g. highly contrived or empty. Assimilations of this kind are familiar and are typically achieved by abandoning the vocabularies normal for describing the assimilated entities and adopting a much more abstract terminology. However, in the present case there is no departure from the normal vocabularies, no such ascent to the abstract. While some rejigging of wording may have occurred in the formulations, the vocabularies throughout are either precisely those of Wittgenstein and Smolensky or, for a few items, uncontentious alternatives. That this is so lends weight to the view that the fact of the similarities is theoretically significant.

Thus, the case mounted in this subsection is as follows. When Wittgenstein's and connectionism's accounts of language mastery are compared, we find that, without departing from the preferred vocabularies, a large number of similarities can be identified, holding without exception between theoretically fundamental, or otherwise significant, features of the accounts, and often between features which have similar structural roles within their respective accounts. This, I conclude, constitutes a substantial case for holding that there is theoretical importance in the existence of these similarities.

A substantial case is evidently not a conclusive case and is always open to the possibility of refutation. In the present instance such a refutation would be forthcoming if it could be shown that a second aspect of the assimilations which Wittgenstein criticizes applied, i.e., if it could be shown that the assimilation had been achieved at the cost of ignoring differences which constitute the theoretically important relationships between the two positions.

Can it be shown that my assimilation of the views of Wittgenstein and connectionism suffers from this weakness? It is not difficult to anticipate arguments that it can and criticisms which I discuss in the next section could be directed to this end. These criticisms turn upon elements of the positions which have yet to be introduced and discussion of them is best postponed. However there is no need to await the introduction of additional views of Wittgenstein or connectionism to anticipate an argument of the kind in question. This is because, in the process of spelling out the very similarities which comprise the assimilation, it was necessary to indicate a general difference between the two positions, one upon which several more specific differences depend.

This allows for an argument that the theoretical importance of this difference is such as to render the fact that there are the similarities I specify theoretically superficial; and that, this being so, any appearance of a substantial case for the theoretical importance of the fact rests upon blindness to the significance of the difference.

The general difference in question, very roughly expressed, is that whereas connectionism's account of linguistic mastery is an account in terms of internal states, Wittgenstein's is an account in terms of public word usage. Several of the similarities I draw attention to presuppose this difference, indeed in the characterizations of the similarities there are ineliminable references to it. Thus to take one of the similarities which turns on the notion of family resemblances, Wittgenstein holds that it is the various public uses of a word which are unified by family resemblances whereas Smolensky holds that it is various representations within connectionist networks which are so unified.

There is no question, therefore, that this general difference (and attendant specific differences) exists between Wittgenstein's and connectionism's accounts; nor that my characterizations of the similarities between them entail that this is so. Moreover, granted the history of debates about the proper account of linguistic mastery or other cognitive accomplishments, there is no question that this difference is of theoretical importance. Thus the issue is at once raised, where does this leave my substantial case for the theoretical importance of the fact of the similarities?

If there is a weakness in my position which turns upon this difference, it clearly cannot be that I make no mention of the difference, nor that I deny that it has theoretical importance. Rather it must be that I am blind to the fact that its theoretical importance is such that it renders the fact of the similarities theoretically superficial. But is there such a fact to which I am blind? My argument that there is not has two stages. First, I shall develop a proposal whereby, far from the theoretical, importance of the difference having this consequence, it is perfectly consistent with the substantial case made out earlier. Secondly, I shall argue for this proposal.

Stated generally the proposal is that the outlined views of Wittgenstein and connectionism are complementary in a theoretically significant way. Their envisaged complementarity may be explained as follows. Wittgenstein's account of language mastery is a descriptive account, a description in terms of salient facts about our usage of ordinary words in a variety of circumstances, about the roles and nature of rules in our everyday usage, about the ways in which language is taught, etc. On the basis of this description he concludes that the symbolic calculus explanation of language mastery is mistaken. But if this explanation is mistaken then there is need of an alternative explanation of language mastery.[3] And if Wittgenstein's descriptive account is correct, then this alternative must explain how it is possible for us to master word usages which are unified only by family resemblances, to follow 'soft' rules, to achieve mastery by teaching methods in which training and examples play essential roles, etc. It is within these assumed constraints that complementarity is proposed. The proposal is that connectionism, in its current state, comprises the early formulations of an alternative explanation of language mastery which can meet these constraints—by 'early formulations' I mean something like the early theories in a Lakatosian scientific research programme.[4] On this proposal, Wittgenstein's descriptive account is construed as a general characterization of the task which an explanatory theory of language mastery must carry out, while connectionism is construed as being engaged in carrying it out through modelling the computational processes which subserve this mastery. So construed the two accounts are complementary and the way in which they are is obviously theoretically significant.

On this proposal the difference referred to earlier is the difference between an account which purports to describe ordinary public

---

[3] I take this to be obviously true but I suspect that some Wittgensteinians may strenuously oppose it. While I very much doubt that Wittgenstein would oppose the idea of an explanation of language mastery of the kind I have in mind, (other than on the grounds that such an explanation is irrelevant to his concerns—see section IV), the issue cannot be addressed here. However, this is an appropriate point to take on board a point made by Andrew Woodfield to the effect that my 'Wittgenstein' may be in disagreement on various points with Wittgenstein. Since I believe in the correctness of the former (though I don't argue this here), it follows that there may be points on which I hold Wittgenstein to be mistaken. Despite this, I would maintain that all the essential views ascribed to Wittgenstein in this paper are his views.

[4] It should be noted that leading connectionists are typically modest in their assessment of the power of current connectionist models. Hinton (1990) effectively expresses the point about the location of current models within a Lakatosian research programme when he writes: 'Most connectionist researchers are aware of the gulf in representational power between a typical connectionist network and a set of statements in a language such as predicate calculus. They continue to develop the connectionist framework not because they are blind to its current limitations, but because they aim to eventually bridge the gulf by building outwards from a foundation that includes automatic learning procedures and/or massively parallel computation as essential ingredients' (p. 2).

features of language mastery and one which is engaged in the task of explaining language mastery thus described in terms of features of internal processing, and such a difference is clearly of theoretical importance. Thus the proposal meets the requirement of acknowledging the difference noted earlier and according it theoretical significance. However, since, on the proposal, the accounts between which the difference holds are significantly complementary, the differences theoretical importance must be consistent with the theoretical importance of the fact that there are many similarities between the accounts. For between significantly complementary accounts there will be many significant similarities and this fact will be theoretically significant. Of course, each of the similarities must be consistent with the difference. While I believe that this can be shown clearly for the similarities I have identified, I shall not attempt to do so here. However, in the following argument for the complementarity proposal, the cases for several of the similarities are implicit. Thus, I conclude that the present proposal shows that the theoretical importance of the difference between the accounts of Wittgenstein and connectionism need not be such as to render the fact of the similarities between them theoretically superficial, i.e. that there need not be any fact in this regard to which I am blind.

But is the complementary proposal correct? In support of the view that it is, I shall, first, present an argument for it and, secondly, defend it against a number of anticipated objections. The remainder of this section will be devoted to the former task, the next section to the latter.

The argument I shall offer here for the complementarity proposal has its source in the proposal's explanatory richness. This explanatory richness is constituted as follows:

(1) As was argued in the first part of this section, there is a substantial case for regarding as theoretically important the fact that there are many similarities between the Wittgensteinian and connectionist accounts. The proposal that the accounts are complementary in the way outlined explains why there are so many similarities, why they possess the other characteristics involved in the arguments which comprise the substantial case, and the nature of the inferred theoretical importance.

(2) The proposal also explains the difference between the accounts, that one describes public word usage while the other describes internal processes, and gives a precise explanation of the evident theoretical importance of this difference.

(3) The occurrence of a broad formal difference among the similarities whereby some are (more or less) agreements (e.g. symbolic

calculus theory is false), whereas the others are not (e.g. the uses of a word on the one hand, connectionist representations on the other, are unified by family resemblances) is explained by complementarity of the proposed kind. Roughly, what connectionism and Wittgenstein reject, and what connectionism explains and Wittgenstein describes, are the very same things, hence the agreements; and, while the connectionist explanation refers to phenomena not mentioned by Wittgenstein, these resemble in certain respects those which Wittgenstein describes, hence the other similarities.

(4) The individual similarities are explained. Here I shall limit myself to significantly different examples. Take a similarity which is an agreement on a positive point, e.g. in learning the meaning of words training with reference to examples plays a central role. This is explained on the proposals that the feature in question is part of the phenomenon of language mastery as described by Wittgenstein and, as such, is a feature which connectionism is engaged in explaining. Or take one of the similarities which is not an agreement, e.g. word usage on the one hand, connectionist processing on the other, are 'soft'. This is explained on the proposals that the 'softness' of word usage is part of language mastery as described by Wittgenstein, and the 'softness' of connectionist processing is part of connectionism's explanation of language mastery which is characterized by 'softness' of word usage.

This explanatory richness is striking. It means that the proposal explains all *prima facie* significant points concerning similarity and difference raised earlier. Relative to these it is a complete explanation. Moreover it is evidently an economical and tightly integrated explanation. Granted these virtues (and the clear absence of a rival proposal with comparable virtues), I conclude that there is a substantial case for the proposal that the views of Wittgenstein and connectionism are complementary in a theoretically significant way.[5]

[5] Clearly, additional arguments are desirable, especially one along the lines that connectionism can be shown to be capable of providing an explanatory theory of language mastery such as Wittgenstein's account requires. As the last footnote and the account of the complementarity proposal imply such an argument is unavailable. However, one could review current connectionist models of language processing for evidence that progress towards this goal is under way, but that would be a substantial undertaking. Moreover, mounting an argument of this kind would seem to render justifiable the demand that a question raised by Stephen Stich should be answered. The question is what one is to make of the fact that the best implementations of models in the Roschian tradition (see Lakoff, 1987), i.e. those which are closest in spirit to Wittgenstein's views on concepts, are symbolic. Evidently these large issues cannot be addressed here.

IV

It is not difficult to envisage objections being raised to the complementarity proposal. The view that Wittgenstein's account of language mastery is complemented by an explanatory account featuring descriptions of connectionist processing will, I believe, strike many as utterly wrong-headed. While it seems to me that there are many grounds upon which a charge of wrong-headedness may be made, it is impossible to discuss them all here. Fortunately many of them may be construed reasonably as forming groups. In this section I shall address three such groups, discussing a representative member in each case. I shall argue that none of these charges are justified and that, indeed, an investigation of two of them serves to deepen and strengthen the complementarity proposal.

Members of the first group have their source in remarks by Wittgenstein of the order that his 'considerations could not be scientific ones' (1958, § 109, cf. p. 230), that he has no interest in scientific hypotheses about cognition (1958, § 156, p. 220), that neurophysiological explanations are irrelevant to his problems (1958, p. 212, cf. p. 216, § 157), etc. To represent this group I shall propose the objection that since connectionism's concern is a scientific explanation of language mastery, and since Wittgenstein's concern is a perspicuous representation of the use of our words to which scientific explanations are irrelevant, the resulting accounts cannot be significantly complementary.

While it is obvious that the concerns of Wittgenstein and connectionism are quite different, it is equally obvious that this mere difference in concerns does not entail that the resulting accounts cannot be complementary. Moreover, the complementarity proposal does not require that either position shares or even respects the other's concerns. What the proposal requires is that specified views which Wittgenstein arrives at in realizing his concerns are complemented by views which connectionism arrives at in realizing its concerns. And there is nothing in the characterizations of the two concerns which implies that this requirement cannot be met, specifically that connectionism cannot explain our use of words as perspicuously represented by Wittgenstein. Short of additional arguments, therefore, there is no reason to regard criticisms of this kind as threatening the complementarity proposal.

Members of a second group of anticipated criticisms stem from the remarks by Wittgenstein which have led some commentators to (mistakenly) regard him as a behaviourist. Among these I will concentrate upon those which concern that part of his treatment of understanding which gives criteriological status to application. In terms of understanding a word the principal point will be that applying the word correctly has criteriological status. How is this supposed to be problematic for the complementarity proposal? I shall assume that it is held to be incompatible with what I shall take to be an implication of connectionism, viz., that in principle connectionism can provide a new, neurophysiological criterion for understanding a word.[6]

This objection fails for a number of reasons. First, for Wittgenstein application is '*a* criterion of understanding' (1958, § 146, my emphasis), not the sole criterion. Secondly, on his conception, a criterion is neither a necessary nor sufficient condition. Thirdly, there is reason to believe that he accepts the possibility of new, neurophysiological criteria for psychological concepts. Certainly the notion of the emergence of new criteria as such is integral to his conception of language as a developing historical phenomenon. More specifically, he discusses the introduction of 'a new . . . physiological . . . criterion for seeing' and his point is not that this is impossible but that it 'can screen . . . from view, but not solve' the conceptual problem which is his concern (1958, p. 212). Finally, the criteriological status of application is virtually implicit in connectionist methodology, whether in the description of tasks to be modelled or in judging the adequacy of a model. Hence this objection (and, I believe, others of its family), far from having force against the complementarity proposal, leads to recognition of further similarities between the positions.

The final group of objections centres upon a presumption about connectionism, viz., that it is reductionist about cognitive theory so that given cognitive kinds are identical to certain neurophysiological kinds. A representative objection is: on account of its reductionism, connectionism holds that understanding a given word is being in a certain neurophysiological state; however, it is fundamental to Wittgenstein's account of understanding that understanding is not a state; therefore, the two accounts of linguistic mastery are incompatible on a crucial point and cannot be complementary.

[6] On Smolensky's interpretation connectionism does not model cognition at the neural level, rather at the higher subconceptual level. However, while it follows that a unit in a model should not be taken to represent a neuron, it is held to represent a real functional entity in the brain, e.g. certain groups of neurons. This seems sufficient to justify my use of 'neurophysiological' here and subsequently. On a later argument I employ, it is perhaps unlikely that connectionism will provide new criteria for understanding words. However it would seem to be a mistake to rule these out in principle.

A possible reply to this objection involves granting that, for Wittgenstein, understanding a word is not a state: for him it is nothing but an ability or capacity to use a word correctly. Secondly, it involves challenging the reductionist reading of connectionism—connectionism is to be understood as holding, not that understanding a word is identical to a certain neurophysiological state, rather that it is an ability or capacity to use the word correctly and that an associated neurophysiological state is the ground of the ability. While this reply neatly defends the complementarity proposal and, I believe, has *some* merit, it should be rejected. Effectively, it condones misinterpretations of both Wittgenstein and connectionism contained in the objection, misinterpretations which prevent recognition of further important similarities between the positions. I shall support this claim in the remainder of this section.[7]

To begin with a crucial point, the objection's implication that Wittgenstein denies that understanding a word is a state is simply false. Wittgenstein unequivocally asserts: '"Understanding a word": a state' (1958, p. 59, insert (a)). What he undoubtedly denies is that understanding a word is a *mental* state, where depression, excitement, and pain are examples of mental states (ibid.). The assertion is sufficient to dismiss the objection as it stands, while the denial is one with which connectionism can concur. However, the question remains of what kind of state Wittgenstein holds understanding a word to be.

Since he denies that it is a mental state there is perhaps a temptation to conclude that he holds it to be a neurophysiological state, a temptation which may be increased by the absence of any unequivocal claim to the contrary. Moreover, in *Philosophical Grammar* the following passage occurs:

> If knowledge is called a 'state' it must be in the sense in which we speak of the state of a body or of a physical model. So it must be in a physiological sense or in the sense used in a psychology that talks about unconscious states of a mind-model. Certainly no one would object to that (1974, p. 48).

Here the example is knowledge, but in his discussion of understanding in *Philosophical Investigations* Wittgenstein frequently notes or implies the close relationship between 'knows' and 'understands' (e.g. §§ 139, 147, 150). Further, the *Philosophical Grammar* passage is embedded in a discussion with striking points of agreement with that in *Philosophical Investigations* in which the

---

[7] I am grateful to Colin Radford for forcing me to clarify and defend the following interpretation of Wittgenstein.

assertion that understanding a word is a state occurs. One point of agreement is that while knowledge and understanding may be called states 'one still has to be clear that we have moved from the grammatical realm of "conscious states" into a different grammatical realm' (1974, p. 48). Another is that the difference between these 'realms' is marked by different employments within them of the term 'continuously'. On the basis of these considerations, then, one may be tempted to conclude that, for Wittgenstein, understanding a word is a neurophysiological state, a view which would bring him into agreement with connectionism as characterized in the objection. Nevertheless, I believe that one should resist this temptation; also, that this being so does not imply any incompatibility with connectionism.

I shall approach my substantiation of these claims indirectly by considering passages in *Zettel* in which Wittgenstein focuses upon what he calls the 'prejudice in favour of psychophysical parallelism' (1981, § 611). An example of this prejudice is that 'there is [a] process in the brain correlated . . . with thinking; so that it would be . . . possible to read off thought-processes from brain processes' (1981, § 608). Wittgenstein professes that no 'supposition seems to [him] more natural than that' psychophysical parallelism is false (ibid.). He makes it clear that in saying this he does not mean to be taken as espousing Cartesian dualism (1981, § 611). What he does mean, he says, is this:

> if I talk or write there is, I assume, a system of impulses going out from my brain and correlated with my spoken or written thoughts. But why should the *system* continue further in the direction of the centre? Why should this order not proceed, so to speak, out of chaos? (1981, § 608)

Before considering the relevance of these remarks to the view that for Wittgenstein understanding a word is a neurophysiological state, I shall discuss their bearing upon the complementarity proposal. On first acquaintance they may seem to run quite counter to connectionism and hence point to a significant weakness in the complementarity proposal. What I propose to argue, however, is that, far from this being so, reflection upon connectionism in the light of the remarks makes it possible to strengthen and deepen the proposal.

First, the idea that a spoken or written thought (or the correlated impulses going out from the brain) could 'proceed, so to speak, out of chaos' is one which it would be natural to ascribe to connectionism—a point which Georges Rey also seems to note (Rey, 1988). According to connectionism, the processing from which the

spoken or written thought proceeds is of the kind which only connectionism is capable of describing exactly and completely.
However, while connectionism can thus in principle give a
description of such processing, it is generally incapable of offering
a tractable explanation of the spoken or written thought.
Generally, tractable explanations must be left to alternative higher-
level formalisms but ones which can yield, at best, rough approxi-
mations or metaphors (Smolensky, 1988). Thus, from the perspective of theories offering tractable accounts—which is the implied
perspective of psycho-physical parallelism—connectionism is perceived as representing cognitive activities as 'proceed[ing], so to
speak, out of chaos'.

Moreover, it should not be thought that all that this entails is
that, for connectionism, the accurate description of the brain
process with which a given thought is correlated is a complex,
microlevel description. What the 'chaotic' character of processing
within a connectionist network entails is that it may well be the
case that, in principle, there is no non-arbitrary way of isolating a
functionally discrete process, within the pattern of activity distributed across the network, which one can say is the brain process
correlated with a given thought. It is possible, of course, to employ
a variety of analytical techniques to reveal differing forms of order
within the 'chaos' but, arguably, these do not provide a non-arbitrary means of individuating a process of the kind psychophysical
parallelism requires. Connectionism, that is, can be plausibly read
as entailing that it is a prejudice to suppose that there is any such
process. Therefore, comparison of the Wittgensteinian and connectionist positions on the topic of psychophysical parallelism
reveals further similarities between them and serves to strengthen,
rather than threaten, the complementarity proposal. The question
which must be addressed, however, is what relevance this conclusion has to the issue of identifying understanding a word with a
neurophysiological state.

In *Zettel* Wittgenstein's remarks concern thoughts. There is no
obvious reason for supposing that they would not apply equally to
what many would be happy to term instances of occurrent understanding of a word. However, this is not the point I wish to make
(and not only because Wittgenstein denies that the mental processes in such cases are instances of understanding). The point, rather,
is that since Wittgenstein denies that there need be a neurophysiological process in the case of the relatively simple phenomenon of
having a thought, it is deeply implausible to suppose that he would
identify the highly complex phenomenon of understanding a word
with a neurophysiological state. Moreover, the same is true of con-

nectionism.

For Wittgenstein, understanding a word involves being able to use the word in many different ways which are inherently open to extension and addition. And, implicit in what I have said earlier about its methodology, the same is true for connectionism. This ability is evidently highly complex and plastic. Granted the earlier points concerning 'chaos' and functional discreteness in the case of thoughts, the proposal that either position would identify what involves this ability (presumably, on the proposal, explains it) with a neurophysiological state cannot be treated seriously. Such a proposal merits application (with minimal adjustment) of Wittgenstein's remark in the *Brown Book*:

> There is a kind of general disease of thinking which always looks for what would be called a mental state from which all our acts spring as from a reservoir (1969, p. 143).

From the connectionist point of view the metaphor is equally inappropriate. Reservoirs are tractably describable and relatively discrete entities while their three dimensional character stands in stark contrast to one of the most useful aids for thinking about connectionist learning, viz., multi-dimensional abstract space (Churchland, 1989).

Thus one should not suppose that since Wittgenstein asserts that understanding a word is a state, but denies that it is a mental state, he holds that it is a neurophysiological state. But in that case, what kind of state can he possibly hold it to be? And is his view compatible with connectionism?

In suggesting answers to these questions I shall commence with a remark from *Zettel*.

> States: 'Being able to climb a mountain' may be called a state of my body. I say: 'I can climb it—I mean I am strong enough' (1981, § 675).

One important point about this remark is that it shows that Wittgenstein does not regard abilities and states as mutually exclusive. This point can be used to make swift progress in answering the first question. For since Wittgenstein calls understanding a word a state, it can be asked whether he also holds it to be an ability or capacity. And the familiar answer to this is that his remarks either imply that he does or that he holds that there is a very close relationship between understanding and ability/capacity (e.g., 1958, §§ 150, 151, p. 181). Thus an answer to the first question is forthcoming: Wittgenstein holds understanding a word to be a state of the kind where a state is an ability or capacity. The ability or capacity in question is, of course, to use the word correctly.

This answer, I believe, is fine so far as it goes, but does not go far enough. What is missing can be gleaned from the *Zettel* passage. The utterance 'I can climb it—I mean I am strong enough' is clearly intended to illustrate the claim that 'being able to climb a mountain' may be called a state of my body. But it also serves to explain the sense in which, on the occasion of this utterance, the ability is a state. And, since the point pertains to 'States', it also serves to explain the sense in which, generally, an ability is a state. What is missing, therefore, in the earlier account of what kind of state Wittgenstein holds understanding a word to be is a specification (or specifications) of the sense in which this ability is a state.

In Wittgenstein's example the ability to climb a mountain on a particular occasion is a state in the sense that the ability consists in being of a certain strength—being of a certain strength constituting a state of the body. On another occasion, where, say, the Matterhorn is the mountain in question, the comparable utterance may be 'I can climb it—I mean I have the specialized skill.' In that case the ability is a state in the sense that it consists in being attuned in a specialized way—being attuned in a specialised way constituting a state of the person. The case of understanding a word is similar to this second example. The ability to use a word correctly is a state in the sense that it consists in being attuned in a specialized way.

The attunement in which the ability to use a word correctly consists can, in principle, be specified several different ways (albeit partially, granted the open-ended nature of the ability). It can be specified in terms of what it is an attunement to do, in which case the specification will be a complex Wittgensteinian-style account of the correct uses of the word in various circumstances. Or, in principle, it can be specified in terms of the details of the dispositions of the internal dynamical organization which the process of attunement has brought about and which enable the word to be used in the ways detailed in the other kind of specification. Effectively, connectionism promises a specification of the second kind and, if it is forthcoming, it will be a highly detailed and complex description of network dispositions couched in terms of units, weightings on connections, and principles of dynamical interaction. Such a specification would evidently complement a specification of the first kind, hence the complementarity proposal is strengthened rather than weakened by consideration of the final objection.

To return to that objection, the preceding discussion implies that it is mistaken on several key counts. Wittgenstein does not deny that understanding a word is a state, rather he holds that it is a state of a particular kind. Connectionism does not hold that understanding a word is a neurophysiological state, rather that it is a state of a different kind, an attunement which constitutes an ability to use a word in myriad ways. Of course, a detailed connectionist specification of the network dispositions comprising the attunement will make reference to neurophysiological states but the understanding is no one or no collection of these. Thus the objection is deprived of both its premises. The first reply to the objection, which I outlined and then dismissed, is also mistaken on several counts. It accepts the mistaken interpretation of Wittgenstein, hence, when it rightly introduces Wittgenstein's view that understanding a word is an ability, it is incapable of reaching the correct interpretation that it is also thereby a state. With respect to connectionism, it rightly sees that connectionism can regard understanding a word as an ability. However, it mistakenly supposes that there is some neurophysiological state to which connectionism is committed and which must be theoretically located as the ground of the ability. Consequently it fails to see that connectionism can regard understanding a word as both an ability and a different kind of state. The reply which I offer avoids all of these mistakes, is firmly based upon Wittgenstein's remarks (including those which are problematic for other readings), involves a plausible reading of connectionism which complements the reading of Wittgenstein, and thus lends further weight to the complementarity proposal.

V

The central claim of this paper is that the views of Wittgenstein and connectionism are complementary in a theoretically important way, the claim I have called the complementarity proposal. In briefly concluding the paper I comment on the claim's virtues.

The claim has a number of virtues. Two of these are detailed in this paper, viz., its explanatory richness (section III) and its capacity to survive serious objections and gain further explanatory power in the process (section IV). However, there is, I will suggest, a third, more general virtue. This is to contribute to and perhaps help broaden the effort, currently manifest in various forms and numerous works, to move beyond what Bechtel and Abrahamsen (1990) have dubbed 'the Exclusively Propositional Era'. If there really is to be a successor era then its ramifications will spread far further than the field in which, understandably, the contemporary effort is most vigorous, viz., that which seeks to establish the nature of the processing which subserves cognitive activities. Moreover, if an integrated theory is to emerge the various manifestations of the effort need to ultimately complement each other. The central claim of this paper can be viewed as holding that two major contributions to this effort do so complement each other and that in combination they display some of the further ramifications mentioned earlier.[8]

[8] I believe that the topics treated in this paper are only some of those raised by non-classical approaches within cognitive science which can be fruitfully addressed within a Wittgensteinian framework. It would hardly be surprising if this were so granted the comprehensive critique in Wittgenstein's later philosophy of the classicist presuppositions and commitments of his own earlier work.

References

Bechtel, W. and Abrahamsen, A. A. 1990. 'Beyond the exclusively propositional era', *Synthese*, **82**, 223–253.

Churchland, P. M. 1989. *A Neurocomputational Perspective: The Nature of Mind and the Structure of Science*. Cambridge, Mass.: The MIT Press.

Hinton, G. E. 1990. 'Preface to the Special Issue on Connectionist Symbol Processing', *Artificial Intelligence*, **46**, 1–4.

Lakoff, G. 1987. *Women, Fire, and Dangerous Things: What Categories Reveal about the Mind*. Chicago: The University of Chicago Press.

Mills, S. 1990. 'Smolensky's interpretation of connectionism: the implications for symbolic theory', *Irish Philosophical Journal*, **7**, 104–118.

Mills, S. 1992. 'On the proper treatment of eliminative connectionism', *Network: Computation in Neural Systems*, **3**, 5–13.

Rey, G. 1988. 'Sanity surrounded by madness', *Behavioral and Brain Sciences*, **11**, 48–50.

Smolensky, P. 1987. 'The constituent structure of connectionist mental states: A reply to Fodor and Pylyshyn', *The Southern Journal of Philosophy*, 26 Supplement, 137–161.

Smolensky, P. 1988. 'On the proper treatment of connectionism', *Behavioral and Brain Sciences*, **11**, 1–23 and 59–70.

Smolensky, P. 1991. 'Connectionism, constituency, and the language of thought', in B. Loewer and G. Rey (eds), *Meaning in Mind: Fodor and his Critics*. Oxford: Blackwell.

Wittgenstein, L. 1958. *Philosophical Investigations*, Second Edition, trans. G. E. M. Anscombe. Oxford: Blackwell.

Wittgenstein, L. 1969. *The Blue and Brown Books*, Second Edition. Oxford: Blackwell.

Wittgenstein, L. 1971. *Tractatus Logico-Philosophicus*, Second Edition trans. D. F. Pears and B. F. McGuinness. London: Routledge and Kegan Paul.

Wittgenstein, L. 1974. *Philosophical Grammar*, trans. A. Kenny. Oxford: Blackwell.

Wittgenstein, L. 1981. *Zettel*, Second Edition, trans. G. E. M. Anscombe. Oxford: Blackwell.

Levels of Description in Nonclassical Cognitive Science

TERENCE HORGAN AND JOHN TIENSON

David Marr (1982) provided an influential account of levels of description in classical cognitive science. In this paper we contrast Marr's treatment with some alternatives that are suggested by the recent emergence of connectionism. Marr's account is interesting and important both because of the levels of description it distinguishes, and because of the way his presentation reflects some of the most basic, foundational, assumptions of classical AI-style cognitive science (*classicism*, as we will call it henceforth). Thus, by focusing on levels of description, one can sharpen foundational differences between classicism and potential non-classical conceptions of mentality that might emerge under the rubric of connectionism.

We say 'potential conceptions' of mentality because at present there is no such thing as 'the connectionist conception of the mind', in the form of a determinate set of foundational assumptions differing in specific, explicit, ways from those of classicism. There may be several, incompatible conceptions of mind that could develop from or be wedded to connectionism. At present, connectionism is primarily an alternative say of *doing things* in cognitive science, rather than an alternative set of doctrines or theses. One constructs network models and trains them up with learning algorithms, rather than writing programs.

We will 'genericize' Marr's three levels of description, yielding a tripartite levels-typology that remains neutral about key foundational assumptions of classicism that are built into Marr's original formulation. With this generic typology as a guide, we will set forth a succession of approaches to mentality which, although they all conform to the generic format, deviate increasingly from classicism.

Each of these approaches could potentially get articulated and defended in the context of connectionist work in cognitive science—although none is necessarily tied to connectionist-style network structures *per se*. The final approach we will describe—the one which differs most radically from classicism—is the one we think probably embodies the truth about human cognition. We will not attempt to argue this here, however; we have done so elsewhere. Our main purposes at present are to propose a map of the intellectual landscape of possible views about mentality, and to *call attention* to several options on that landscape that have been largely overlooked—not only by philosophers, but also by practising cognitive scientists, connectionists included.

1. Marr's Three Levels

Marr suggests that in order to understand complex information-processing systems, qua processors of information, one needs to consider such systems from a tripartite theoretical perspective. He writes:

> At one extreme, the top level, is the abstract computational theory of the device, in which the performance of the device is characterized as a mapping from one kind of information to another, the abstract properties of this mapping are defined precisely, and its appropriateness and adequacy for the task are demonstrated. In the center is the choice of representation for the input and output and the algorithm to transform one into the other. At the other extreme are the details of how the algorithm and representation are realized physically—the detailed computer architecture, so to speak (1982, pp. 24–25).

He labels these three levels, respectively, (1) the theory of the computation; (2) representation and algorithm; and (3) hardware implementation.

The top level involves systematic transitional connections among intentional state types as such. For a cognitive system as a whole, these are *total cognitive states* (TCS's), sometimes comprising several individual cognitive states that are simultaneously co-instantiable (perhaps in various different cognitive subsystems). The theory of computation delineates a *cognitive transition function* (CTF) over TCS's. For all TCS's instantiable by the system, the CTF specifies the appropriate immediate-successor TCS's. The CTF is the function to be computed by the system.

The middle level involves the account of how cognitive transitions are subserved by computation. This level addresses the kinds of structured states that serve as representations, and the computational processes by which these representations are manipulated. These processes conform to programmable rules that are purely formal, i.e., that advert solely to the form or structure of the representations and not to their content. The formal rules over the representations constitute an *algorithm* for computing the CTF; i.e., under the relevant assignment of content to the representations, processing in conformity to the rules is guaranteed to effect the cognitive transitions described by the theory of the computation.

The level of implementation, in turn, involves the account of how the formal/syntactic representations are themselves subserved by physico-chemical states and structures, and how the rule-describable manipulations of these representations are subserved via physico-chemical causal processes.

Within classical cognitive science, theorizing at Marr's top level typically involves a whole vertical hierarchy of sub-levels. In terms of familiar flow-chart analyses ('boxology', as Cummins (1983) puts it), one adds another, lower, sub-level by adding more inter-connected boxes to one's flow chart, either between existing ones or within them. Each box in a flowchart depicts a specific function that gets computed, within the system. The entire flowchart, for a total cognitive system, depicts the system's CTF; thus the system's TCS, at any moment t, is the full set of inputs and outputs (at t) to and from each box in the overall flowchart. Elaborating the flowchart, by adding additional boxes within or between the current ones, is essentially the boxological counterpart of hypothesizing that the system computes the functions represented by the boxes in the original flow chart by computing compositions of other functions—where the compositions are depicted by the more detailed boxology. (The function f is a composition of the functions g and h if $f(x) = g[h(x)]$) The system thus computes each CTF in the hierarchy *by* computing a more fine-grained CTF in which its embedded. Impressive cognitive transitions are thus ultimately composed of numerous cognitive 'baby steps', many of which are presumed to be rapid and unconscious. Each of these baby steps is simple enough to be subservable by symbol manipulation conforming to rules that advert only to the syntactic structure of the symbols, not to their content. Choice of symbol forms and rules adverting to those forms moves one to Marr's middle level.

For both Marr's top (cognitive-transition) level and his middle (algorithm) level, the downward inter-level relation between (i) state-types at that level, and (ii) state-types at the level just below it, is evidently the relation commonly called *realization*. How best to characterize the realization relation is a metaphysical question beyond our concerns in this article. But two key features of the relation bear emphasis. First, it is transitive: if a state-type S realizes a state-type R, and R in turn realizes a state-type T, then S realizes T. Second, it is a many-one relation: in general, a realizable state-type is *multiply* realizable by a variety of different lower-level state types[1].

Philosophers and cognitive scientists undoubtedly think of the relation between Marr's middle level and his bottom level as realization, in the sense just characterized. Indeed, Marr's term 'implementation', which he invokes to name the bottom level, is essentially the computer scientist's word for what philosophers call realization. But among philosophers at least, it has not always been appreciated that the relation between Marr's top and middle levels is also best viewed as realization; there has been a tendency to instead construe the latter as *type identity*. Yet the case for realization as the top/middle bridging relation is quite straightforward, and goes as follows. Since a single computable function can generally be computed by a variety of distinct algorithms (some employing different representations than others), there is bound to be a one-many relation between (i) the cognitive transition function at the Marr's top level, and (ii) the algorithms (with their associated representations) that compute that function. But middle-level state-types are individuated functionally, in terms of the specific algorithms in which they figure; distinct algorithms yield distinct middle-level state types. Hence, the intentional mental states posited by the theory of the computation are multiply realizable at the middle level, by various different computational state-types.[2]

As he presents it, Marr's tripartite account seems to build in the

[1]Multiple realizability is no doubt ubiquitous in nature. The case most discussed is higher-level state-types being differently realized in different species or creature-kinds. But the same higher-level state-type might be multiply realizable in different members of the same species; or in a single individual at distinct moments in its own history; or even in a single individual at a single moment in its own history.

[2]For further elaboration of this point, see Horgan (1992). Marr himself evidently saw the point quite clearly—as evidenced in the following passage from Marr (1977). The passage sets forth an example to illustrate the distinction between the computational level of description and the algorithm level, in a way that also brings in the hardware/wetware level: [T]ake the case of Fourier analysis. The (computational) theory of the Fourier transform is well understood, and is expressed independently of the particular way in which it is computed. There are, however, several algorithms for implementing the Fourier transform—the Fast Fourier transform ..., which is a serial algorithm, and the parallel 'spatial' algorithms that are based on the mechanisms of coherent optics. All these algorithms carry out the same computation, and the choice of which one to use depends upon the available hardware. In passing, we also note that the distinction between serial and parallel also resides at the algorithm level and is not a deep property of a computation' (Marr 1977, p. 37).

assumption that human cognitive processing is deterministic at the intentional level of description. For, what a computational system computes is a *function* from TCS's to TCS's; and such a function pairs each TCS with a unique TCS as its successor. (Marr's immediate concern was to provide theoretical underpinnings for his own computational theory of vision, which was deterministic at the cognitive level.) But classical cognitive science can, and often does, allow for non-deterministic cognitive transitions. And it can, and often does, apply the notion of computation to the middle-level processes that subserve such transitions.

It is not difficult to generalize Marr's characterization of the three levels of description in classicism, to explicitly accommodate non-deterministic cognitive transitions and 'non-deterministic computation'. The basic idea is essentially this: the middle-level processes still count as computation because they still conform to programmable rules over representations; it's just that these rules include occasional 'dice throws' (involving, say, the system's consulting a random-number table), with subsequent processing steps depending on the outcome of the dice throws.[3]

2. Foundational Assumptions of Classicism

The classical view that cognition is mathematically realized by an algorithm, i.e., by rule-governed symbol manipulation, involves three basic assumptions:

(1) Intelligent cognition employs structurally complex mental representations.

[3] In keeping with the classical idea that cognition is computation, this means generalizing the notion of computation in some appropriate way. We suggest one way of doing it in Chapter 2 of Horgan and Tienson (forthcoming a). The reader should keep in mind, for the discussion that follows, that classicism allows for the possibility that a human CTF is non-deterministic, and that the notion of 'computing' a TCS should be understood accordingly. (A non-deterministic CTF is a function that takes each CTF to the *set* of its potential successor TCS's or to a probability distribution over the members of that set.)

Note that in this passage he uses the term 'implementation' to characterize the relation between the computational level and the algorithm level. The idea is that computations are implemented via algorithms, which themselves get implemented in hardware (or wetware); multiple modes of implementation are possible between each level and the one immediately below it.

(2) Cognitive processing is sensitive to the structure of these representations, and thereby is sensitive to their content.
(3) Cognitive processing conforms to precise, exceptionless rules, stable over the representations themselves and articulable in the format of a computer program.

Claims (2) and (3) are frequently not distinguished at all or are taken to be equivalent. But it is crucial to avoid this conflation; (3) implies (2), but (2) does not imply (3). This becomes important in Sections 7 and 8, below.

We will call the rules mentioned in (3) *programmable, representation level, rules* (for short, PRL rules). It is important that these rules are supposed to be stable at the level of the representations themselves; i.e., they refer solely to those structural aspects of the representations that play representational roles. Although processing in certain systems may also conform with rules stable at one or more lower levels (e.g., the level of machine language in a conventional computer), such lower level rules are not the kind that count. This is important because there can be (non-classical) systems that conform to programmable rules at lower levels, but do not conform to rules stable only at the level of representations, as we discuss in Section 8, below.

Classicism does not assert that the PRL rules of cognitive processing must be represented by (or within) the cognitive system itself. Although programs are explicitly represented as stored data structures in the ubiquitous general purpose computer, stored programs are not an essential feature of the classical point of view. Rather, a classical system can conform with representation-level rules simply because it is hardwired to do so. It is, for example, plausible from the classical point of view to regard some innate processes as hardwired.

Assumptions (1)–(3) are widely recognized. However, to assert that cognitive transitions are subserved by an algorithm that computes those transitions is to presuppose something further, something so basic that its status as an assumption is often not even noticed, viz.,

(4) Human cognitive transitions conform to a tractably computable function over total cognitive states (TCS's).[4]

[4] The commonly heard term 'tractably computable' is vague and perhaps also somewhat context dependent. '*Not* tractably computable' means something stronger, of course, than simply not *easily* computable. 'Not tractably computable' seems sometimes to be used to mean something like: not computable with the computational resources that are available or likely to become available. It also seems to be used with a—

This is hardly a truism; on the contrary, it is a very strong assumption indeed. Even granting that human cognitive transitions conform to a function, there is nothing independent of the assumptions of classicism to indicate that the cognitive transition function must be computable, let alone tractably computable. However, this assumption is never, to the best of our knowledge, argued for on independent grounds.

It is obviously presupposed by classicism, since cognitive transitions couldn't possibly be subserved by computation unless those transitions were themselves tractably computable.

With respect to assumptions (1)–(4), an attitude of 'What Else Could Cognition Be?' has pervaded classicism since its inception. The intended force of the rhetorical question is that there is nothing else it could be. Cognitive states have content-based causal roles, and it is felt that the only way they could have such roles is via computational processes. The question is rhetorical, but taken literally as a question it is fair enough; below we will sketch some answers.

Assumptions (1)–(4) of classicism are built right into Marr's tri-level typology for cognitive science. But classicism makes an additional foundational assumption, which is not officially presupposed in the three levels as characterized:

(5) Many mental representations encode propositional information via language-like syntactic structure.

Although classicists can, and sometimes do, allow that *some* computational processes subserving human cognition might operate on representations with some kind of formal structure other than language-like syntactic structure, they also maintain that the systematic semantic coherence of human thought rests largely, and essentially, on computational manipulation of language-like mental representations.

3. Genericizing Marr's Three Levels

Marr's tri-level typology for cognitive science is a species of a more generic tri-level topology. Table 1 describes both versions:

not unrelated—sense something like: not computable with roughly the order of computational resources of the human brain, whatever that may be. It does not matter for our present purposes which sense is used. To overcome the vagueness of the term, when we discuss below the possibility that human cognitive transitions do not conform to a tractably computable function, we will mean that they do *not* do so under any reasonable resolution of the vagueness of 'tractably computable'.

Table 1

	Marr	*Generic*
Top level:	COGNITIVE FUNCTION	COGNITIVE STATE-TRANSITIONS
Middle level:	ALGORITHM	MATHEMATICAL STATE-TRANSITIONS
Bottom level:	IMPLEMENTATION	IMPLEMENTATION

The generic version will serve as a touchstone below when we describe some potential alternatives to classicism.

Notice, to begin with, that Marr's three levels conform to this more generic characterization. A cognitive function will determine cognitive state-transitions. And the theory of algorithms is, of course, a part of mathematics. An algorithm, or program, is a mathematical beast, a set of rules for manipulating symbols or data-structures purely on the basis of their formal/structural properties, independently of any intentional content they might have; and the symbols and data-structures, so described, are themselves mathematical objects.

Cognitive science, since its inception, has embodied the following central and important idea about cognitive design, an idea reflected both in Marr's own typology and the generic one. What is important about the brain, *vis-à-vis* mentality, is not its specific neurobiological properties, but rather the abstract functional/organizational properties in virtue of which the physical state-transitions are systematically appropriate to the content of the mental states they subserve. These properties involve neither physical states and structures *qua* physical, nor mental states and structures *qua* mental; they are mathematical. The mathematical level of description is the appropriate one for characterizing the abstract system of functional/organizational features that constitutes Nature's engineering design for human cognition. This level mediates between the other two: cognitive states are realized by mathematical states, which in turn are realized by physical states of the cognizer's hardware or wetware.

The seminal idea that a system of mathematical state-transitions is the locus of cognitive design is built into classicism, with its emphasis on the algorithm. The genericization of Marr's three levels retains this key idea, but does so without building in assumptions (1)–(5) of classicism. There is more to mathematics, of course, than those branches of it that have traditionally figured most prominently in computer science. Part of what's important about connectionism is the mathematics that goes most naturally with it. We turn next to that.

4. Connectionist Networks and Dynamical Systems[5]

If one focuses on the theoretical and mathematical aspects of the recent connectionist movement in cognitive science, one finds connectionists increasingly invoking a rich mathematical framework with a distinguished history: the mathematical theory of *dynamical systems*. This framework fundamentally involves *continuous* mathematics rather than *discrete* mathematics—even though it can be brought to bear on systems which, at the relevant level of description, are literally discrete (say, because they evolve in discrete time-steps). In classicism, on the other hand, discrete mathematics is the natural mode of description: computation, as investigated in logic and computability theory, is the discrete, stepwise, rule-governed manipulation of symbols and data structures. An algorithm, or a program, is a set of rules for such discrete symbol manipulation.

To treat a system as a dynamical system is to specify in a certain way its temporal evolution, both actual and hypothetical. The set of all possible states of the system—so characterized—is the system's abstract *state space*. Each possible state of the system is a point in its state space, and each magnitude or parameter is a separate dimension of this space. The dynamical system, as such, is essentially the full collection of temporal trajectories the system would follow through state space—with a distinct trajectory emanating from each possible point in state space. A dynamical system can be identified with a set of state space trajectories in roughly the same sense in which a formal system can be identified with the set of its theorems. Just as there are many different axiomatizations of a formal system such as S5 or the classical propositional calculus, so likewise there might be many different mathematical ways of delineating a certain dynamical system or class of dynamical systems. (It is common practice to use the term 'dynamical system' ambiguously for abstract mathematical systems and for physical systems—such as planetary systems and certain networks—whose behaviour can be specified via some associated mathematical dynamical system. In the present paper, we will use the term mainly for mathematical systems.)

[5]This section is largely adapted from section 3 of Horgan and Tienson (1992a).

In classical mechanics, for instance, the magnitudes determining the state space of a given mechanical system are the instantaneous positions, masses, and velocities of the various bodies in the system. Temporal evolution of such a system, from one point in its state space to another, is determined by Newton's laws, which apply globally to the entire state of the system at an initial time.[6]

An *attractor* in state space is a point, or a set of points, in state space toward which the system will evolve from any of various other points. These others are said to lie within the *basin* of the attractor—the idea being that the attractor itself lies at the 'bottom' of the basin. The *boundary* of an attractor basin separates those points in state space lying within the basin from those lying outside it. A *point* attractor is a single stable point in state space; when a system evolves to a point attractor, it will remain in that state (unless perturbed). A *periodic* attractor is an orbit in state space that repeats back on itself; when a system evolves to a periodic attractor, it will oscillate perpetually through the same sequence of states (unless perturbed). A *quasiperiodic* attractor is an orbit in state space which, although it is not literally periodic, is asymptotic to a periodic trajectory. A *chaotic* (or *strange*) attractor is a nonrepeating orbit in state space that is not quasiperiodic. (Chaotic attractors are probably important in the brain's information processing. See Skarda and Freeman (1987), and Freeman (1991).)

A dynamical system is a geometrical/topological sort of mathematical critter. A useful geometrical metaphor for dynamical systems is the notion of a *landscape*. Consider a system involving just two magnitudes; its associated state space is two dimensional, and thus can be envisioned as a Cartesian plane. Now imagine this plane being topologically molded into a contoured, non-Euclidean, two dimensional surface. Imagine this 'landscape' oriented horizontally, in three dimensional space, in such a way that for each point p in the system's two dimensional state space, the path along the landscape that a ball would follow if positioned at p and then allowed to roll freely is the temporal trajectory that the network itself would follow, through its state space, if it were to evolve (without perturbation) from p. A dynamical system involving n distinct magnitudes can be thought of as a landscape too; it is the

[6]Some dynamical systems, including many that have been studied in physics, evolve in accordance with relatively *simple* laws, typically involving global states of the system. Usually such laws are expressed via differential equations, or difference equations if discrete time-steps are involved. But it is very important to appreciate that in general, a dynamical system need not conform to such laws.

n-dimensional analog of such a two dimensional, non-Euclidean, contoured surface: i.e., a topological molding of the n-dimensional state space such that, were this surface oriented 'horizontally' in an (n+1) dimensional space, then a ball would 'roll along the landscape', from any initial point, in a way that corresponds to the way the system itself would evolve through its state space (barring perturbation) from that point.

Connectionist systems are naturally describable, mathematically, as dynamical systems. The magnitudes determining the state space of a given connectionist system are the instantaneous *activation* levels of each of the nodes in the network. Thus the state space of a network is frequently called its 'activation space'. The activation space of a network has as many dimensions as the network has nodes. The rules governing the system's temporal evolution apply locally, at each node of the system; this simultaneous local updating of all nodes determines the system's evolution through time.[7] The topology of a given network's activation landscape will be jointly determined by two factors: (i) the structural features of the network, in particular the pattern of connections between nodes and the weights on these connections; and (ii) the rules by which the individual nodes update their own activations and output signals. In connectionist models, cognitive processing is typically construed as the system's evolution along its activation landscape from one point in activation space to another—where the initial point in the temporal trajectory, and also the final point, and perhaps certain intermediate points, have certain representational contents (whereof more presently). In typical systems a problem is posed to the system by activating a set of nodes which are interpreted as having a certain content. From a dynamical systems perspective, this amounts to positioning the system at some point in its state or activation space. (Which specific point this is will often depend also upon the activation level of nodes other than those involved in posing the problem.) The network eventually settles into a stable state which constitutes its 'solution' to the problem—another point in its activation space. From the dynamical systems perspective, the system has evolved to a point attractor, from an initial point—the posed problem—within the associated attractor basin.

Learning too is typically construed, within connectionism, as temporal evolution of a connectionist network through a state space. When the issue is learning as opposed to processing, howev-

---

[7] Thus, connectionist networks need not, in general, conform to simple update-rules expressible over global activation-states. Cf. note 6.

er, the weights on the network's connections are viewed as malleable rather than fixed; learning involves incremental changes in the weights. Hence the relevant states of the system are given by total specifications of its weights, at a given moment of time during learning. From the dynamical systems perspective, learning is thus a matter of the network's temporal evolution through its *weight space* (with the weight of each inter-node connection being a dimension of this space). However, a connectionist network as it evolves through weight space is not by itself a full-fledged dynamical system, because weight changes are effected not by the network itself, but by system-external application of a weight change algorithm.

Henceforth in this paper, we will frame our discussion with an eye toward connectionist networks as the sorts of physical devices that are to subserve cognitive processing. For simplicity, our focus will be on cognitive processing in a fixed network, rather than on learning; since the relevant dynamical systems will thus be ones whose dimensions correspond to activation levels of individual nodes, we will frequently refer to such a mathematical system as an 'activation landscape'.

Also for simplicity, we will couch our remarks in terms of *entire* connectionist networks, and the entire activation landscape subserved by a given network. But it should be kept in mind that a total connectionist network can consist of distinct, though interacting, subnetworks; and hence can be mathematically analysed as subserving separate, though coupled, dynamical systems. At the mathematical level of description, in such a case, the component dynamical systems are embedded in a larger, higher-dimensional, total dynamical system—just as the component physical sub-networks are embedded in a larger total network.

Though we focus on connectionism for concreteness, our discussion below is not necessarily limited to connectionist systems *per se*. Human-like cognition might only be subservable by physical systems quite different in nature from current connectionist networks; and in principle, our subsequent discussion would carry over, *mutatis mutandis*, to such alternative systems. Moreover, it is probably a mistake to treat the notion of a connectionist system as determined by the sorts of networks currently being explored under the rubric of connectionism. In a broader sense, a 'connectionist system' might better be construed simply as any dynamical system, physically realized by a network architecture. In this broader sense, there are numerous possible connectionist systems (including human brains, perhaps) that differ substantially from the kinds of networks currently being explored by connectionists.

Several points about connectionist systems as dynamical systems should be borne in mind, with respect to the remarks to follow. First, we again stress that the dynamical system, the activation landscape, is not itself a *physical* system; rather, it is a high-dimensional *mathematical* entity, a topologically complex surface in a high dimensional space. This space is not directly, but indirectly and abstractly, related to the physical space of the network that realizes it.

That is, second, although this abstract entity is indeed physically realized by a network, local regions of the activation landscape will not, in general, correspond to physically local portions of the *network*; quite the contrary. A *point* in activation space is determined by activation values for *every* node in the network; i.e., by the network as a whole. Conversely, a given value for a single node in an n-node network determines an n−1 dimensional region of activation space.

Hence, third, the more physically distributed the scheme of representation—so that representations are physically subserved by activation patterns involving many nodes, rather than by activation in single nodes or small node-pools—the more efficiently the abstract space is used for realizing representational states; i.e., the more physically distributed the representations, the more abstractly local! If representation is relatively local physically, so that relatively few nodes are required to take on certain values in order for a given TCS to be realized, then numerous total activation states of the system will realize that TCS; and each of these total activation states corresponds to a different point in activation space. Conversely, if representation is highly distributed, then in general comparatively fewer points in activation space will count as realizers of the TCS. In the extreme case of distributed representation, a TCS is realizable only by a single total activation pattern over all the nodes of the network; mathematically, the corresponding activation vector specifies a *unique* point in activation space.

Fourth, as dramatic recent developments in the mathematics of dynamical systems have shown, physical systems in nature can realize dynamical systems involving enormously complex, and enormously non-homogeneous, variation in local topography at different local regions of the abstract temporal landscape.[8] (This

[8]This is especially true when the physical systems involve nonlinear dynamical behaviour. Connectionist networks are like this, as they provably must be to avoid well known limitations in their computational power similar to the limitations of two-layer perceptrons. Each node updates its activation in accordance with a non-linear function.

local topological complexity can involve, among other factors, the nature of the attractors, including chaotic ones; the nature of the basin boundaries, including fractal ones; and highly intricate inter-twinings of attractor basins, some of them fractal.) Hence, fifth, the more distributed the scheme of representation, and hence the more localized the representational states are in *abstract* space, the greater are the opportunities for harnessing this local topological complexity, on the abstract activation landscape, to subserve sophisticated cognitive processing.

5. Connectionist Systems as Implementation Architecture

With the discussion in Sections 1–4 as groundwork, we turn now to a succession of potential approaches to mentality that all fall under the generic tri-level typology of Section 3, and yet differ in increasingly radical ways from classicism. We will proceed 'up from the bottom' through the three levels. In this section, without yet calling into question classicism's assumptions about mathematical transitions or about cognitive transitions, we consider connectionist networks as potential implementations the classical conception of cognition. Then in Section 6 we will turn to the view that the mathematical transitions, although they do involve algorithmic manipulation of representations, employ only representations whose formal/mathematical structure is *non-sentential*. In Section 7 we will consider the possibility that human cognition is mathematically subserved by a (network-realizable) dynamical system that is *non-algorithmic*. Finally, in section 8 we will consider the possibility that human cognitive transitions do not conform to a tractably computable function at all.

The dynamical-systems mathematical framework is quite broad and general, and is not intrinsically incompatible with the classical theory of computation. In principle, a connectionist network might be characterizable both (i) as executing an algorithm over representations, and (ii) as realizing a certain dynamical system. That is, mathematically, the network would subserve *both* an algorithm for computing a cognitive transition function, *and* a dynamical system whose trajectories through its state space subserve that function. If so, then in terms of the three levels of description from Section 3, the algorithmic characterization would belong to the mathematical level, whereas the dynamical-system characterization would belong to the implementation level. For, the latter would specify, albeit mathematically rather than physically, one way among many of implementing the algorithm—a way that is itself physically realizable via a network structure.[9]

So the least radical possibility for connectionism is that it might provide for new ways of implementing computational processes over structurally complex mental representations, including language-like representations. This might lead to interesting new developments at higher levels of description—for instance, to new kinds of algorithms, ones that are more naturally implemented in connectionist architecture than in von Neumann machines. Important as such new developments might be, however, they would not amount to a new conception of cognition, over against classicism's conception. On the contrary, as long as assumptions (1)–(5) from Section 2 remain in force, cognition is still being conceived classically. Implementational connectionism would be no deviation from classicism at all, but merely a species of it.[10]

6. Non-Syntactic Computationalism

One way to depart from classicism, however, is to reject assumption (5), while still retaining (1)–(4). On this view of the mind, human cognitive transitions do conform to a tractably computable transition function over total cognitive states; and these transitions

[9]This way of putting the point involves seeing the implementation level as hierarchically stratified, involving one or more mathematically specified sub-levels before 'bottoming out' in physical states and state-transitions in a physical machine. This kind of implementational hierarchy is ubiquitous in conventional computers: there is a mathematically describable 'virtual machine', executing algorithms over sentences that belong to a high-level formal language and whose content is the information the system is supposed to be processing; this mathematical machine is simulated by another mathematically describable machine, executing algorithms over sentences in a different formal language whose sentences have different representational content (typically, some sort of number-crunching content); this simulational embedding of one mathematical virtual machine within another proceeds down to the level of machine language, and then bottoms out in physical realization of the lowest-level mathematical machine.

One could, alternatively, think of the hierarchy as belonging to the middle, design level, and the implementation level as involving only physical realization. However one chooses to put it, the point is that there is typically an implementational hierarchy between the level of cognitive design and bottoming out in physical realization.

[10] Cf. Fodor and Pylyshyn (1988). For a more detailed discussion of the matter of 'mere implementation,' see Horgan and Tienson (1992b).

are still subserved by an algorithm that computes that function— i.e., by PRL rules over mental representations. However, the representations themselves are not sentential, and thus their structure is not *syntactic* structure.

With connectionist networks in mind one might claim, for instance, that mental representations are non-sentential *vectors*, and that the algorithm effects vector-to-vector transformations that are systematically sensitive to vectorial structure, and thereby are systematically sensitive to the content of these non-sentential representations. Connectionist networks, on this view of things, are devices that are naturally suited to perform such non-sentential computation; vectors are realized as activation patterns over sets of nodes. Thus, the claim goes, connectionism can and should evolve toward non-sentential computationalism as an alternative to classicism.[11]

This approach fits naturally, although perhaps not inevitably, with the idea that human cognition, at the top level of description, involves state-transitions that are all essentially *associative*—in the sense that they reflect statistical correlations among items the cognitive system can represent, and can be analysed as the drawing of statistical inferences. Many fans of connectionism evidently see things this way, and tend to regard connectionism as breathing new life into associationism. Prominent foes of connectionism, notably Fodor and Pylyshyn (1988), also see things this way; but they regard the link with associationism as grounds for maintaining that connectionism, in so far as it strives to do more than implement classicism, is bound to founder on the same kinds of problems that plagued traditional associationism. Concerning the non-implementational prospects for connectionist networks in cognitive science, Fodor and Pylyshyn write:

> A good bet is that networks sustain such processes as can be analysed as the drawing of statistical inferences; as far as we can tell, what network models really are is just analog machines for computing such inferences. Since we doubt that much of cognitive processing does consist of analysing statistical relations, this would be quite a modest estimate of the prospects for network theory. (p. 68)

We ourselves share Fodor and Pylyshyn's doubts about the prospects for associationism, given the problems this doctrine

---

[11]Paul Churchland (1989) is a fan of connectionism who appears to see the matter this way.

faces in accommodating the semantic coherence of thought. On the more general question whether human cognitive transitions conform to a transition function that is tractably computable via computational processes operating entirely over non-sentential representations, we are also pessimistic; again, it is hard to see how rule-based transformations of representations could reflect the systematic semantic coherence of thought, for the vastly many distinct cognitive states that humans are capable of instantiating, unless many of those representations encode propositional information in systematic, productive ways, i.e., syntactically.

More fundamentally, however, we doubt whether cognition in general is subserved by representation-level computation *at all*— i.e., that it is subserved by transformations of representations in accordance with PRL rules.[12] Still more fundamentally, we doubt whether human cognitive transitions even conform to a tractably *computable* transition function, either a deterministic one or a non-deterministic one. Connectionism, we think, might well be weddable to non-classical conceptions of mentality that are more radical than non-sentential computationalism, and that have little to do with associationism. It is time to turn to these.

7. Non-Algorithmic Dynamical Systems

Perhaps human cognitive transitions are subserved by a dynamical system that is not also an algorithm for computing those transitions. Even if human cognitive transitions happen to be tractably computable, as classicism assumes, they might not be subserved via representation-level computation—i.e., via manipulation of language-like mental representations, in conformity with PRL rules adverting to the structure of those representations. Instead, the system's transitions from one total cognitive state to another might leap fairly large cognitive gaps in single steps that are not decomposable, via classicist 'boxology', into computationally subservable cognitive baby steps (either serial ones, or simultaneous

---

[12]It is the PRL rules we doubt, not the representations; this is why we have elsewhere called our view 'representations without rules.' We also maintain that human cognition requires representations with some form of *syntax*. But if the proper middle level of description in cognitive science involves a dynamical system and not an algorithm, as we believe, then syntactic constituency relations are likely to look very different than in classicism. See the end of Section 7, below.

ones, or both).[13] This possibility, obviously, is quite radically at odds with classicism.

Here is a simple hypothetical example, to illustrate what we mean. Consider standard decision theory, viewed as a putative psychological model of human deliberation and choice, rather than a normative theory. According to this model, a deliberating agent will choose an action with maximum expected utility. The expected utility of an envisioned act is a certain kind of weighted sum: the sum of the respective numerical values the agent assigns to the various envisioned potential outcomes of that act, with each value being weighted by the agent's subjective probability of the given outcome's resulting from the act.

Now, one way that such a decision-making system might work would be computational. For instance, it might actually *calculate* this weighted sum, for each envisioned act; then compare the totals for the acts and *calculate* which act or acts have maximal expected utility; and then pick an act with maximal expected utility. But here is another possibility, without representation-level computation. There are various beliefs and desires at work in the system, with various strengths. They all enter the hopper at once and interact directly—somewhat in the manner of a complex combination of interacting physical forces in a planetary system, with the various bodies exerting mutual gravitational influence on one another. The way they interact is via a kind of 'resolution of forces', where the forces get resolved in such a way that the cognitive system eventually settles on an alternative with maximal expected utility.[14]

Under this second mode of mathematical realization, there would be no separate baby steps (either sequential or simultaneous) of actually calculating weighted sums, of actually comparing them pairwise, and the like. Instead there would be a mathemati-

---

[13]The metaphor of connectionist systems leaping large cognitive gaps in a single bound is from Lloyd (1991). He there floats, as worth serious consideration, the limit-case view that all mental states are conscious ones—there are no unconscious, intervening mental steps between conscious mental states.

[14]The analogy with the interaction of physical forces is not exact, since the cognitive system must settle into *cognitive* states, and in general a relatively small portion of the physical states of the system will realize cognitive states. (Equivalently, only relatively few points in activation space realize cognitive states.) Simple summation of forces in a network would in general not lead to cognitive states. Thus, there must be some sort of 'winner-take-all' feature built into the cognitive system that ensures that it ends up in cognitive states (and by and large, relevant ones).

cally more direct route to a decision: viz., the system's *settling*, by evolving quickly and automatically to a point attractor realizing a decision to go with one of the acts that has maximal expected utility. One of the potential acts *wins out*.

It is important to appreciate that this hypothetical scenario would indeed constitute a very important departure from classicism. At the mathematical level of description, we would have not an *algorithm* that subserves cognitive transitions via representation level computational baby-steps (either sequential or simultaneous), but instead a dynamical system that subserves cognitive transitions via non-algorithmic, leaps-and-bounds-ish, state transitions.[15]

It is also important to realize that connectionist networks could, in principle, subserve non-algorithmic cognitive transitions, even though each node in the network updates its own activation, locally, in accordance with an algorithm. For, the local updatings of individual nodes need not be parallel baby-steps in some algorithm *over representations*—some set of programmable rules for manipulating and transforming complex representations on the basis of their representation-level structure. Instead, the node-level computation in the network might be entirely *sub*-representational, and hence implementational. This possibility seems especially salient for connectionist systems in which activation-levels of individual nodes do not have any specific, determinate, representational content—for instance, systems employing a representation scheme in which all representations, even the semantically atomic ones, are *distributed* activation-patterns.

The example of a non-algorithmic decision maker is hypothetical. We turn now to an actual connectionist model which is a good *prima facie* candidate for being a system that performs a sophisticated information-processing task in a non-algorithmic way. It is a model of natural-language sentence parsing, due to George Berg (1992).[16] The system receives, as external input, a temporal sequence of word-representations, each of which represents a suc-

---

[15] With non-algorithmic dynamical systems, in general one might expect there to be many fewer cognitive transitions than are posited in classicism, because classical models often require numerous sequential cognitive baby-steps (many of which are supposed to occur rapidly and unconsciously); cf. note 13 above. When the temporal trajectory subserving a cognitive transition passes through a number of intermediate points on the activation landscape, it may be that few or none of those points realize *cognitive* states.

[16] The task is sophisticated enough that it probably cannot be accomplished by a purely associative/statistical algorithm, one that merely per-

cessive word in an English sentence. It constructs a representation of the sentence's syntactic structure; and it can recursively decompose this parse-representation, in order to successively represent the sentence's main syntactic constituents, then the main sub-constituents of each of these constituents, and so on—all the way down to the constituent words.

Berg's model adapts and extends an approach for representing recursive structures first developed by Jordan Pollack (1990), called 'recursive auto-associative memory', or RAAM. In Pollack's RAAM networks, the representations all have so-called 'fixed bandwidth'; i.e., for any node-pool in which representations are instantiated, each representation is a fully distributed activation pattern involving every node in the pool. In one part of a RAAM system, fixed-bandwidth representations can be constructed for recursive structures of arbitrary complexity; in the other part, such representations can be recursively decomposed, thereby successively reconstructing the representations of the successive substructures.

The overall structure of Berg's network is depicted in *Figure 1*. It has five layers, with recurrent feedback from the hidden layer back to the input layer. Nodes are segmented into specific pools, as shown. The input layer has two pools, one for word-representations and the other which duplicates the current hidden-layer representation. The output layer has four pools, one for each of the

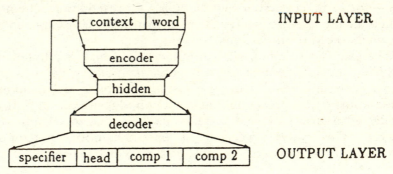

Figure 1. The basic structure of Berg's parser network (Berg, 1992)

forms statistical inferences involving, for instance, transition-frequencies among words of English. And as we discuss below, the network generalizes substantially beyond the English sentences that constitute its training corpus—which means that it presumably doesn't learn by merely encoding a 'look-up table' correlating each input in its training regimen with the correct output. Thus, Berg's model is a plausible candidate for being a system that performs a *non-associative* information-processing task in a non-algorithmic way.

178

four syntactic roles—specifier, head word, first complement, and second complement—of an 'X-Bar template' of the sort posited in the form of theoretical syntax known as 'government and binding theory' (cf. Chomsky 1981, Sells 1985). Such X-Bar structures can exhibit recursive embedding, because the roles of specifier, first complement, and second complement can be filled by X-Bar structures themselves.

Representations in Berg's model are fixed-bandwidth activation patterns. Words get represented as distributed activation patterns in the word pool of the input layer, and in the head-word pool of the output layer. These two pools have the same number of nodes, this number being the bandwidth of the word-representations. X-Bar structures themselves, including the 'null' structure, get represented as distributed activation patterns in the hidden layer, in the context pool of the input layer, and in the specifier and complement pools of the output layer. Each of these pools has the same number of nodes, this number being the bandwidth of the X-Bar representations.

Construction of parse representations occurs in the first three layers of Berg's network, in the following way. A representation of the first word of an English sentence is activated in the word pool of the input layer, with the context pool initially dormant; activation then passes forward through the encoder layer to the hidden layer, thereby generating in the hidden layer a tentative, partial, parse representation. This tentative representation is then copied back to the 'context' pool in the input layer, at the same time that the next word of the English sentence is being activated in the 'word' pool; activation then passes forward from the context and word pools of the input layer, through the encoder layer to the hidden layer, thereby generating a new tentative parse representation. This process continues, with as many feed-forward passes from input to hidden layer as there are words in the English sentence. The hidden layer ends up containing a fully distributed representation of the sentence's syntactic structure.

Recursive decomposition of the parse representations occurs in the bottom three layers of the network, as follows. When the total parse representation is present in the hidden layer, activation is fed forward through the decoder layer to the output layer; this generates, within the four respective pools in the output layer, fixed-bandwidth representations of the sentence's four primary X-Bar constituents—the specifier, head word, first complement, and second complement respectively. (Some of these constituents might be null.) If the specifier-representation, and/or either complement-representation, is not null, then it can be copied back into the hidden layer, and then decomposed by another forward activation-pass through the decoder layer to the output layer. This process can be conducted recursively; along the way, fixed-bandwidth representations of all the sentence's syntactic constituents and sub-constituents get recovered. (The atomic constituents, i.e., the words, all turn up at one point or another in the head-word (or specifier) pool of the output layer.)

Since the parse representations all have fixed bandwidth, regardless of the complexity of the parse structures they represent, recursive complexity in the representations themselves is obviously not a matter of parse-substructures being represented by activation patterns that are physical components of the activation patterns representing the larger structures. But recursive information is systematically encoded nonetheless, since the representations of X-Bar sub-structures are recursively recoverable from representations of the larger structures.

Berg trains up his network, as did Pollack his original RAAM systems, by means of a sophisticated adaptation of the back-propagation learning algorithm, incorporating what Pollack calls the 'moving target strategy'. Back-propagation is a method which adjusts the weights of the network in the direction of the correct, 'target' output, doing this repeatedly until the network produces the correct output. Pollack divides the training regimen into successive 'epochs'. With the moving target strategy, in each epoch, the 'target' representations, for whole tree structures and for their constituent sub-structures, are the ones the system itself has developed in the preceding epoch. The representations thus change along with the weights from epoch to epoch, in a process of controlled co-evolution.[17] The system, as it learns, gradually *discovers* appropriate representations. With sufficient training, it gradually converges on a combination of weights and representations under which the representations of parsing structures and substructures are recursively recoverable, accurately and systematically.

Berg's connectionist parser works quite well, on a wide range of sentences of varying recursive depth. It also generalizes quite effectively to new sentences that were not part of the training corpus. Berg writes:

> Testing and training are done on separate corpora each containing the patterns for 1000 sentences. The average sentence is between 6.5 to 7 words long... The corpora contain sequential presentations of randomly generated, syntactically legal sen-

[17]Berg's training procedure implements the moving target strategy somewhat differently than does Pollack; but the differences need not concern us here.

180

tences. There is no restriction on the length or 'depth' of the generated sentences. . . This results in most of the sentences being between 2 and 8 phrases deep, with fewer sentences of greater depths, typically with a maximum between 14 and 20. . . [These] networks typically converge to 1–8% overall error for both training and testing corpora. (p. 5)

From the successive decoding of the phrases of a sentence, one can read off the X-Bar syntax of that sentence. *Figure 2*, for instance, is an 'unrolled network' diagram showing how a series of decodings reveals the overall syntactic structure of a sample sentence.

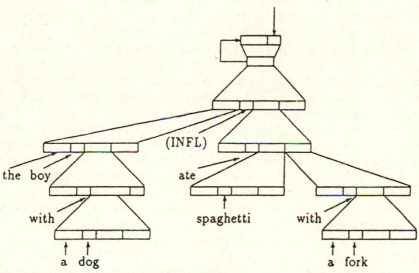

Figure 2. The 'unrolled' network for the sentence 'the boy with a dog ate spaghetti with a fork'. Unlabelled phrases at the output level are empty (Berg, 1992)

It seems highly unlikely that this connectionist system does this parsing by executing an algorithm at the level of representations themselves. There are two interrelated reasons to think so. First, the representations are quite thoroughly distributed: activation values of individual nodes are not assigned any specific, determinate, representational content. Since rules for activation-updating apply locally at individual nodes, whereas representation is fully non-local, the node-level computations appear to be purely sub-representational, rather than being component steps in some set of (highly parallel) representation-level rules. Second, although the structures being represented have varying, arbitrarily deep, recursive complexity, all such structures are represented by activation patterns of the *same* bandwidth, within the *same* pools of nodes;

hence, recursive complexity of representational content is quite unrelated to the physical part/whole structure of the representations themselves. Since the activation patterns representing complex structures are not anything like 'physical sums' of smaller activation patterns representing the component sub-structures, it is all the more unlikely that the system's manipulation of these patterns can be analysed as conforming to PRL rules involving numerous simultaneous representation-level baby-steps.

But how else, it might be asked, *could* the system be accomplishing its parsing task so successfully, if not by implementing some representation-level algorithm? What other sort of characterization might it have, at the mathematical level of description, that would constitute a successful design for the subserving of systematically content-appropriate transitions over intentional states?

Part of what we find interesting and exciting about Berg's model, and also about Pollack's RAAM's, is that their use of the 'moving target' training strategy suggests a general answer to this question: an alternative, non-classical, approach to mathematical design for information-processing systems. The key ideas are as follows. As the network gets progressively altered at the physical level during learning, via successive changes in the weights on the connections, at higher levels of description what's happening is the progressive co-evolution of two interrelated factors. On one hand, the dynamical system itself is being altered by weight changes; the local topography throughout the high-dimensional activation landscape is being progressively *molded*. On the other hand, because of the moving target strategy, there is also progressive alteration of the position of representations on the activation landscape.[18] This repositioning effects a refinement of the realization relation from intentional states (i.e., representational states qua representational) to points on the activation landscape. The realization relation exhibits increasing systematicity, coming to reflect, in the way it positions representation-realizing points relative to one another on the activation landscape, important relations among the intentional states being realized. The realization relation and the landscape topography end up 'made for each other', with respect to the information-processing task the system is being trained to perform: the final weight setting

[18]At the physical level of description, intentional states are realized in networks by activation patterns. But mathematically, the activation vector describing a particular physical pattern is also a specification of a set of coordinates in the dynamical system's state-space. Thus, from the dynamical systems perspective, the states realizing a given intentional state are the points on the activation landscape that have the coordinates specified in that vector.

for the network subserves a high-dimensional activation landscape whose overall local topography yields systematically content-appropriate temporal trajectories, under the operative intentional/mathematical realization relation. Thus, the key to the system's design is that the shape of the activation landscape, and the overall positioning of representation-realizing points on that landscape, are jointly just right to subserve the relevant intentional transition function, for a very large class of potential intentional states. Moreover, it's neither an accident nor a miracle that this is so; rather, it's the understandable result of applying a learning algorithm in a way that incorporates the moving target strategy.

There is nothing in this story about cognitive design that requires that a cognitive system even conform to programmable rules over representations, let alone proceed by executing such rules. This story evidently is true of Berg's system. So we have a possible answer to the question: how else, if not by a representation-level algorithm, could the system accomplish its parsing task?

In addition, the story is obviously quite general in its potential scope: it is entirely possible that the abstract 'engineering design' for much of human cognition does not involve any representation-level algorithm, but instead involves a high-dimensional activation landscape and a cognitive/mathematical realization relation that fit together like hand and glove to subserve the system's cognitive transition function. For a human, of course, the CTF involves an *enormous* range of distinct total cognitive states the system can instantiate—vastly more than it ever *will* instantiate in its lifetime. Given this fact, and given that all trajectories on the activation landscape that commence from any TCS-realizing point must yield content-appropriate cognitive transitions, a suitable cognitive/mathematical realization relation would probably have to exhibit a very high degree of systematicity: i.e., it would position all the TCS-realizing points throughout the landscape in such a way that their various relative-position relations reflect many important semantic relations among the TCS's themselves.

The semantic relations reflected in this way would very likely include relations of *semantic constituency* among complex intentional states: for instance, the relation *being about the same individual*, or the relation *predicating the same property*. In so far as (i) such semantic constituency relations get systematically reflected in the positioning in activation space of representation-realizing points, and (ii) this fact is important in the dynamical system's successfully subserving content-appropriate cognitive transitions, these relative-position relations would function as *syntactic* relations. That is, the overall distribution of representation-realizations in high-dimensional activation space would structurally encode the kinds of semantic relations that get encoded in public languages by names, predicates, quantifiers, and so forth; and would do so in a manner that is directly implicated in the design whereby the system subserves cognition—and in particular is directly implicated in the explanation of the systematicity of cognition that Fodor *et. al.* have rightly insisted on. This is not what Fodor and McLaughlin (1990) call *classical* syntax, by which they mean a kind of structural constituency in which the constituents of a complex representation are always tokened whenever the representation itself is tokened. It is, however, the kind of syntax that looks natural for an approach to cognitive design in which cognition is subserved, at the mathematical level of description, by a dynamical system rather than an algorithm over representations.[19]

8. Cognition without (Tractable) Computability

Classicism's most fundamental foundational supposition, the one we listed as assumption (4) in Section 2, is that human cognitive transitions conform to a tractably computable transition function (CTF) over total cognitive states (TCS's)—either a deterministic function or a non-deterministic one. As yet we have not questioned this assumption. The burden of Section 7 was that even if it is true, classicism might be mistaken anyway. For, human cognitive transitions might be subserved not by an algorithm that computes the CTF, but rather by a non-algorithmic dynamical system.

It is very important, however, that the general approach to cognitive engineering just sketched does not *presuppose* that a human CTF is tractably computable. Thus arises an even more radically non-classicist possibility: viz., that a human CTF is not a tractably computable function at all, either deterministic or non-deterministic. A CTF that is not tractably computable might be subservable by a non-algorithmic dynamical system which is itself subservable by a neural network.[20]

[19] Some might object to calling relations of relative position, among points in activation space, syntactic constituency relations, even though they do reflect relations of semantic constituency in a way that figures centrally in the system's design. We ourselves think that this usage is indeed sanctioned by the ordinary, pre-theoretical notion of syntax. But the important question, of course, is whether the relative-position relations *can* play this role—not whether their doing so would suffice to sanction calling them syntactic.

[20] Most of what we say in this section applies if a human CTF is not computable at all—which may be the case if there are literally infinitely

What would it mean for a human CTF not to be tractably computable? In addressing this question, it is useful to think about ways the function might, or might not, be specifiable. The CTF itself can be construed as an enormous set of ordered pairs, each of which associates a single TCS with a set of one or more successor TCS's. One way to specify this function would be via a huge (possibly infinite) *list*: each ordered pair in the CTF being specified by a separate entry on the list. Such a list, even if finite, would be truly gargantuan—far too big to itself constitute a tractable set of programmable rules.[21] So to be tractably computable, given the enormous number of distinct cognitive transitions, a CTF would have to be fully specifiable in some way other than via a brute list.

What classicism assumes, of course, is that a human CTF is specifiable via some set of *general* laws over cognitive states; each cognitive transition is just a particular instance of these laws, and the function the laws delineate is itself tractably computable. Conversely, if the CTF is not tractably computable then it will not be thus specifiable. If cognitive transitions are effected by a dynamical system of the sort imagined in the previous section, there is no reason why the CTF would have to be tractably computable.

This would not necessarily mean that there would be no interesting, systematic, psychological laws. For, there remain these two possibilities: either (i) there are psychological laws that fully specify the CTF, but happen to delineate a transition function that is not tractably computable; or (ii) there laws that only *partially*

---

[21]This is our answer to the main argument of Aizawa (forthcoming). To get a sense of how huge the list would have to be, there are on the order of 10^{20} English sentences of 20 words or less (Miller 1965). For most of these there is a potential corresponding thought, and potential thoughts far outstrip sentences because of our ability to make relevant discriminations that we lack linguistic resources to describe. For comparison, there are 10^{10} or so neurons in the human brain, and there have been around 10^7 seconds in the history of the universe.

---

many distinct cognitive states that a cognizer can instantiate. If there are only finitely many such states, then the cognizer's CTF is computable in the official mathematical sense. We take no stand on whether there are literally infinitely many cognitive states that human cognizers can instantiate, or only a huge finite number. Our view is that if human CTF's are computable at all in the mathematical sense, it is only because they are finite. But *tractable* computability is the important concept in the context of classical cognitive science, so we will focus on this.

185

specify the CTF, because they contain ineliminable *ceteris paribus* clauses adverting to potential psychology-level factors that could prevent *ceteris* from being *paribus*.[22]

In general, the failure of a CTF to be tractably computable could be the result of either or both of the following factors: (i) the dynamical system itself, whose mathematical state-transitions might not be tractably computable; or (ii) the way TCS's are realized as points in the dynamical system's state space. Concerning the first factor, it may well be possible for non-computable dynamical systems to be subserved by neural networks—especially if the networks are made more analog in nature by letting the nodes take on a continuous range of activation values, and/or letting them update themselves continuously, rather than by discrete time steps.

Moreover, even if the mathematical state-transitions of the dynamical system are tractably computable (as they are, for instance, for current connectionist systems—which are usually simulated on standard computers), the CTF subserved by the dynamical system might fail to be tractably computable anyway. Consider the converse of the realization relation between TCS's and points in a dynamical system's state-space. This is a function—call it the *realizes-function*—mapping points in a dynamical system's state space to TCS's. (It is a function because it never pairs a point in state space with more than one TCS.) This function itself might not be tractably computable. If not, then obviously it would not be possible to compute cognitive transitions this way: given the initial mathematical state of the dynamical system, (i) compute the dynamical system's trajectory through state space; and (ii) for each point p on the trajectory, compute the TCS (if any) realized by p. And if the cognitive transitions subserved by the dynamical system are not computable in *this* way, it seems likely that they would turn out not to be tractably computable in any other way either. That is, there might well be a network-subservable dynamical system S, a CTF C, and a realizes-function R, such that

(i) S's mathematical state-transitions are tractably computable;
(ii) C is not tractably computable; and yet
(iii) S subserves C, under R.

Needless to say, therefore, one should not infer from the fact that a system's non-cognitive state transitions are tractably com-

---

[22] The second possibility is the one we ourselves think most likely for human cognizers. Cf. Horgan and Tienson (1989, 1990, forthcoming a).

putable that it cannot subserve a CTF which fails to be tractably computable.

The possibility that cognitive transitions are not tractably computable deserves to be taken very seriously. Given what we have said in the last two sections, tractably computable CTF's might well be only a rather small subset of the CTF's that nature could have evolved the hardware to subserve. Thus there is no obvious reason to suppose that nature's CTF's *are* tractably computable.

Moreover, we have elsewhere argued (Horgan and Tienson 1989, 1990, forthcoming a, forthcoming b) that when one reflects carefully on certain problems (like the frame problem) that have persistently arisen in classicism and that largely spawned connectionism, a strong case emerges for the contention that human cognition is just too complex and too subtle to conform to programmable representation-level rules. If so, then the heart of Nature's evolutionary blueprint for human cognition cannot be an algorithm; instead it might well be a non-algorithmic dynamical system, subserving cognitive transitions that are not tractably computable at all.

References

Aizawa, K. forthcoming. 'Representations without rules, connectionism, and the syntactic argument', *Synthese*.

Berg, G. 1992. 'A connectionist parser with recursive sentence structure and lexical disambiguation', *Proceedings of the American Association for Artificial Intelligence*, in press.

Chomsky, N. 1981. *Lectures on Government and Binding*. Dordrecht: Foris.

Churchland, P. M. 1989. *A Neurocomputational Perspective: The Nature of Mind and the Structure of Science*. Cambridge, MA: M.I.T. Press.

Cummins, R. 1983. *The Nature of Psychological Explanation*. Cambridge, MA: M.I.T.

Fodor, J. A. and Pylyshyn, Z. 1988. 'Connectionism and cognitive architecture: a critical analysis', in S. Pinker and J. Mehler (eds) *Connections and Symbols*. Cambridge, MA: M.I.T. Press.

Fodor, J. and McLaughlin, B. 1990. 'Connectionism and the problem of systematicity: why Smolensky's solution doesn't work', *Cognition, 35*, 183–204.

Freeman, W. 1991. 'The physiology of perception', *Scientific American, 264*, 2, 78–85.

Horgan, T. 1992. 'From cognitive science to folk psychology: computation, mental representation, and belief', *Philosophy and Phenomenological Research, 52*, 449–84.

Horgan, T. and Tienson, J. 1989. 'Representations without rules', *Philosophical Topics,* **17**, 27–43.

Horgan, T. and Tienson, J. 1990. 'Soft laws', *Midwest Studies in Philosophy* **15**, 256–79.

Horgan, T. and Tienson, J. 1992a. 'Cognitive systems as dynamical systems', *Topoi,* **11**, 27–43.

Horgan, T. and Tienson, J. 1992b. 'Structured Representations in Connectionist Systems?', in S. Davis (ed.) *Connectionism: Theory and Practice.* Oxford: Oxford University Press.

Horgan, T. and Tienson, J. forthcoming a. *Connectionism and the Philosophy of Psychology: Representational Realism without Rules.* Cambridge, MA: M.I.T. Press.

Horgan, T. and Tienson, J. forthcoming b, 'A nonclassical framework for cognitive science', *Synthese.*

Lloyd, D. 1991. 'Leaping to conclusions: connectionism, consciousness, and the computational mind', in T. Horgan and J. Tienson (eds), *Connectionism and the Philosophy of Mind.* Dordrecht: Kluwer.

Marr, D. 1982. *Vision.* New York: Freeman.

Marr, D. 1977. 'Artificial intelligence—a personal view', *Artifical Intelligence* **9**, 37–47. Reprinted in J. Haugeland (ed.) *Mind Design,* Cambridge, MA: M.I.T.

Miller, G. 1965. 'Some preliminaries to psycholinguistics, *American Psychologist,* **20**, 15–20.

Pollack, J. 1990. 'Recursive distributed representations', *Artificial Intelligence,* **46**, 77–105.

Sells, P. 1985. *Lectures on Contemporary Syntactic Theories.* Stanford, CA: Center for the Study of Language and Information.

Skarda, C. and Freeman, W. 1987. 'How brains make chaos in order to make sense of the world', *Behavioral and Brain Sciences* **10**, 161–95.

Systematicity in the Vision to Language Chain*

NIELS OLE BERNSEN

1. Introduction

Connectionism seems likely to have come to stay as a second computational paradigm for cognitive science in addition to the paradigm of classical AI (for the latter, see, e.g., Pylyshyn 1984). Connectionism with distributed representations throughout has been proposed as a complete, self-sufficient and non-hybrid alternative to the classical paradigm in accounting for the representational states and processes of cognitive systems, biological or otherwise (Smolensky 1988, Smolensky *et al.* 1992). However, just as the general term 'connectionism' continues to lack a clear definition as an alternative computational paradigm for cognitive science, there still remains fundamental unsolved problems for *distributed* connectionism to serve as such a general paradigm. These problems concern how to account for the constituent structure of thought and will be addressed in what follows. It is claimed that these problems can be solved both theoretically and in working connectionist simulations. Distributed connectionism, therefore, has a strong claim to being considered a second general computational paradigm for cognitive science.

Fodor and Pylyshyn (F&P, 1988) have argued that thoughts or representational mental states, just like natural language, have *combinatorial syntactic and semantic structure* and that the utilization of such structural properties is crucial to inference and reasoning. It is because mental representations have combinatorial structure that it is possible for mental operations or processes to apply to them by reference to their form. Thus, mental processes have *structure sensitivity*. Structures of expressions can have causal roles because structural relations are encoded (or implemented) by physical properties of brain states in appropriate ways. Localist

*The research was carried out under grants from the Danish Research Councils for the Natural Sciences and for the Humanities. Their support is gratefully acknowledged. I am indebted to the continued help from Ib Ulbæk and Peter Wolff with the System 2 simulations described in this paper.

189

connectionist networks, F&P claim, do not have combinatorial syntactic and semantic structure and the processes operating over them do not have structure sensitivity. Such networks, therefore, are at most vehicles for the implementation of cognition rather than accounts of cognition at the proper theoretical level which according to F&P is the level of complex symbol structures. Distributed representation networks are no better off in this respect than are localist networks, they claim. Briefly, the argument runs as follows with respect to localist networks: such networks need one set of elements to represent, e.g., the thought that John loves Mary and a different set of elements to represent the thought that Mary loves John. No one set of elements is able to represent the combinatorial syntax of the thought that John loves Mary for the simple reason that such a set of elements does not have combinatorial syntactic and semantic structure. In particular, the unit which fires whenever the system entertains the thought that John loves Mary does not have syntactic and semantic constituent structure. It is a simple, atomic and therefore unstructured unit which fires whenever the system has the thought that John loves Mary. And of course, processes involving this unit cannot be sensitive to a structure that the unit does not have.

It is possible to provide localist networks with constituent structure and variable binding (e.g., Ajjanagadde and Shastri 1991). We have done work on localist networks at CCI using a different approach and found such networks significantly more efficient than distributed networks solving the same problems in spatial cognition (Bernsen and Kopp 1993). However, localist networks are implausible from a cognitivist point of view and will not be discussed here. As for distributed networks, the long discussion fuelled by Foder and Pylyshyn's original paper still has not produced clear and stable solutions (Smolensky 1987, Fodor and McLaughlin 1990, Smolensky *et al.* 1992). The present paper attempts to identify some of the reasons why this is so.

The plan for the paper is as follows: Section 2 offers a semi-formal presentation of the systematicity challenge to connectionism. Section 3 defines a first set of criteria which may enable a specific distributed connectionist system to meet the challenge. The system itself, *System 1*, is described in Section 4. In Section 5, a number of objections to System 1 as a satisfactory solution to the systematicity challenge are considered. One of these objections leads to the construction of a new distributed connectionist system, *System 2*, with a rather different architecture and a cognitive task slightly different from that of System 1 (Section 6). The results of a recent simulation done with System 2 are discussed in Section 7 leading to the conclusion that the systematicity challenge has now been fully met. However, a further twist to the argument remains and is discussed in Section 8. The final conclusion (Section 9) is that there is now strong, if not entirely conclusive, reason to leave the systematicity issue alone and carry on with the more substantial issues of cognitive science. Protagonists of the classical position will have to make significant progress to keep the discussion alive.

2. The Systematicity Argument

In a semi-formal expression, F&P's original argument goes like this:

(a) Information-processing which produces intelligent behaviour has a natural sub-class which is called *cognition* and which includes thinking, reasoning, understanding and generating natural language, etc.

(b) Cognition involves thoughts as a form of mental representation.

(c) Thought has a small number of basic properties which we may call *the set P*. The set P includes properties such as:

- systematicity;
- compositionality;
- inferential systematicity;
- and, possibly, other properties which have yet to be discovered.

Comment: The properties included in the set P replace, for the sake of the systematicity argument, the properties of 'combinatorial syntactic and semantic structure' and 'structure sensitivity' noted in Section 1 above. The properties of systematicity and compositionality will be explained under (d) below. The property of (semantic) compositionality will not be discussed separately since nothing in F&P's argument hinges on the possible differences between systematicity and compositionality. It will be evident from the argument below that if systematicity is not a problem for distributed connectionism, neither is compositionality. The property of (some measure of) compositionality follows from systematicity both on F&P's account and on the present alternative account. The property of inferential systematicity will not be discussed separately as it does not form part of F&P's central argument. I shall simply conjecture that if distributed networks can handle systematicity, they can also handle inferential systematicity *using the very same cognitive mechanisms* as they use in handling systematicity.

(d) The units of (localist) connectionist systems have no internal structure. Two units representing the thoughts that John loves Mary and that Mary loves John, respectively, have no common structure (they have no structure). It follows that such systems might be able to have, e.g., the thought that John loves Mary but unable to have the thought that Mary loves John. This possibility shows that such systems are not characterized by systematicity, that is, their ability to think some thoughts is not *intrinsically* connected to their ability to think certain others, even though both sets of thought involve exactly the same concepts or lexical entries and are composed by using exactly the same compositional principles. However, this does not preclude that localist connectionist systems can be crafted to implement classical architectures of cognition. Compositionality, in this context, is simply the fact that the systematically related thoughts that a system is able to have are not only related syntactically but also semantically. That is, which thoughts are systematically related is not arbitrary from a semantic point of view.

(e) Such systems, with or without the capacity for natural language, which lack systematicity, do not exist in nature. In nature, behaviour, thought, output of cognitive modules, and language are necessarily systematic.

Comment: Note that the systematicity argument does not rest on systems' possession of linguistic capacity. We are dealing with a much more fundamental property of thought and mental representation. Non-linguistic animals and infraverbal cognition also demonstrate systematicity of thought and F&P claim that the inadequacy of connectionist models as cognitive theories follows quite straightforwardly from this empirical fact. Basically, the thesis of the systematicity of thought is a claim about the systematicity of representations underlying a great deal of the observable behaviour in humans and animals. If some human or animal is able to think certain thoughts (or have certain mental representations), they are necessarily also able to think certain other thoughts which can be seen to be systematically (or intrinsically) related to the former.

(f) Distributed connectionist systems are not necessarily systematic, or at least have not yet been shown to be so, unless they merely implement classical physical symbol systems. On distributed connectionist principles, the systematicity of thought is a *mystery*, F&P claim. However, they do not claim to be able to prove that distributed connectionist systems are necessarily unable to exhibit systematicity without merely implementing classical cognitive architectures. Rather, the burden of proof is laid on distributed connectionism.

(g) The systematicity argument does not presuppose the physical symbol systems hypothesis (or the classical paradigm for cognitive science).

(h) It follows from (a)–(g) that connectionism cannot (in principle or at least at present) account for thought. Since thought is basic to cognition, connectionism does not constitute an alternative general paradigm for cognitive science. Now, since the physical symbol systems hypothesis *can* account for thought (or the set P), the hypothesis that classical constituents are tokened as part of the thought they syntactically constitute is the 'only game in town' as an account of thought and hence of cognition. Thought has combinatorial syntactic and semantic constituent structure in the sense of the physical symbol systems hypothesis. In particular, distributed connectionist systems are at best implementations of classical cognitive architectures.

I shall accept (a)–(e) and (g) for the sake of the argument, (c), (e) and (g) being accepted with no qualification other than a bracketing of the theoretical motivations behind F&P's notion of thought. The crucial issue, therefore, is (f) to which we may now turn. If (f) is false, the conclusion (h) does not follow.

3. A First Reply to the Systematicity Argument

To show that (f) above is false, it must be demonstrated

- that distributed connectionist systems *are able* to produce systematic mental representations;
- the *cognitive* mechanism(s) which cause this to be *necessarily* the case must be made clear. These mechanisms, of course, cannot and should not be classical syntactic and semantic ones. Otherwise, doubts may remain as to whether what has been produced is merely a connectionist implementation of a classical cognitive architecture.

A crucial assumption in the argument below is that distributed systems do not have classical syntax (or *ditto* constituent structure). Given this assumption, if (f) is shown to be false in the manner just indicated, distributed connectionism can be considered a general paradigm for cognitive science. I shall come back to that assumption in Section 8 below. The claim we are considering is the claim that *only* classical syntax or the existence of an internal syntactic structure of mental representations can explain the systematicity of mental representation that is evident from much of human and animal behaviour.

Clearly, nothing hinges on representing the particular examples concerning John's love for Mary and Mary's love for John. Indeed, 'love' is a very difficult concept to represent, and not only in connectionist systems. We are thus free to choose a different example for experimental demonstration and subsequent interpretation. On the other hand, the issue does seem to be one of representing central cognition or linguistically expressible thought rather than possibly unconscious and linguistically inexpressible peripheral cognitive states.

So we need an example of a complex thought. It could be a two-place, asymmetrical relational thought just like the ones about John and Mary above. The thought should have systematicity in the sense that a system should not be able to have the thought that aRb (or $R(a,b)$) without, necessarily, being able to have the different but systematically related thought that bRa (or $R(b,a)$), a and b representing individuals. If a connectionist system with distributed representations is able to entertain such systematically related thoughts then this system demonstrates systematicity. It also demonstrates compositionality in the rather limited sense of Section 2 above. And, *ex hypothesis*, it does so without having syntactical representations in the classical sense of the term. Finally, we would like to be able to explain why systematicity necessarily obtains in the system.

An example meeting the above constraints is the relational thought partially caused by perception that something (e.g., a triangle, or John) is to the right of something else (e.g., a square, another triangle, or Mary). Let us apply some conditional reasoning to this example:

If a distributed connectionist system

- can learn from experience something which for the sake of the argument is sufficiently close to the concept of 'spatial object in general'; and
- can learn from experience something which for the sake of the argument is sufficiently close to the concept of 'right-of-ness in general' as correctly applying to two arbitrary spatial objects; *then*

- it *does not matter* to the system whether it applies these concepts to R(a,b) which it has seen in the training set, or it applies them to R(b,a) which it has not seen in the training set;
- the system therefore *necessarily* realizes systematicity through a distributed version of variable binding where:
- variable binding is achieved through processes of *abstraction* from experience, *generalization* from experience, and *instantiation* to new, currently experienced instances which it has not seen before; and
- variable binding is dynamically achieved through patterns of weighted connections and without classical syntactic constituency and syntactic combinatorial structure.

Such a system will have other classical properties as well such as an infinite generative capacity (if it could only be tapped in some way), basic context-independence of its representations, and semantic compositionality in the sense of Section 2 above. In fact, the system is in many respects similar to a classical system which might be capable of solving the same cognitive task. The system processes 'real' semantic material which might have been produced by a machine vision front-end and it produces output which might be input for further processing by a natural language generation module. It is therefore consistent with the hypothesis of modular cognitive architecture. Furthermore, the system learns the concepts it has from experience which is undoubtedly the way biological systems come to have such concepts as the ones considered here.

Note that nothing has been said about syntax above. It is not claimed that the described system acquires, through experience and training, a syntactic representation of the form '*right-of(x,y)*'. It is not claimed that, on the basis of such a representation the system performs a formal syntactic operation of binding, through the operation of substitution which we call instantiation, the variables x and y to, say, John and Mary. Such representations and operations form part of one *particular* (i.e., syntactic) algorithmic way of describing what the system might be doing. As hypothesized above, our distributed connectionist system does not do things this way. It does learn the abstract concept that *something* is spatially related to *something else* through the relation 'right-of'. But instead of the variables x and y it has a pattern of weighted connections between its units of activation which perform *as if* they were variables like x and y, or, rather, which perform the same cognitive task as that performed by a syntactic system with variables x and y, but differently. And the distributed system does not formally bind the variables x and y (which it does not have) to the particular individual objects it perceives through the formal syntactic operation of substitution. Rather, the 'something' and 'something else' representations of the network (which are realized by its weighted connections and units of activation) become activated by input representing individual objects in space. This activation allows the network to determine whether or not those objects stand in the right spatial relationship for the relationship 'right-of' to obtain between them.

The system described does not, strictly speaking, know of formal logic and does not represent the world in terms of formal logic. But it does represent abstract concepts and knows how to apply them to individuals that it perceives in its world. It represents abstract concepts of two kinds. First, it represents the concept of a spatial object in general, more or less. Second, it represents the concept 'right-of' in general, more or less, since it is able to correctly describe objects in different positions as being or not being to the right of other objects. The powerful mechanisms of abstraction from experience and subsequent instantiation to experienced objects are what is responsible for these capabilities and thus for the system's mastery of systematicity (and compositionality). The crucial point is that the system does master (non-syntactic) combinatorial semantic constituent structure. In other words, if such a system can be built, it will realize systematicity at the cognitive level through algorithmic means that are basically different from those of classical syntactic systems.

The abstract representation which our hypothesized system has 'that some spatial object is to the right of some other spatial object' would clearly seem to count as a semantically *complex* representation. Being abstract, this representation is, at least in principle, able to *generate* infinitely many different instantiations. In virtue of its abstractness, it is also to a large extent *context-independent* (contrast Smolensky 1988). We obtain these classical properties without having to assume a syntactic level of representation tokening atomic symbols and complex symbols having atomic symbols as their parts.

It turns out not to be too difficult to build a distributed connectionist system with these capabilities. The system is a kind of micro-world animal, but in contrast to the animal described by F&P (1988) this animal masters systematicity: 'Such an animal would be, as it were, *aRb* sighted but *bRa* blind, since presumably, the representational capacities of its mind affect not just what an organism can think, but also what it can perceive. In consequence, such animals would be able to learn to respond selectively to *aRb* situations but quite *un*able to learn to respond selectively to *bRa* situations. (So that, though you could teach the creature to choose the picture with the square larger than the triangle, you couldn't for the life of you teach it to choose the picture with the triangle larger than the square).'

4. System 1

We have built a network with distributed representations having the properties described above (Bernsen and Ulbæk 1992a). The simulated network learned how to apply the concept 'to the right of' through being trained on pictures of discriminably different 2-D objects. A semantic difficulty had to be overcome. The concept 'to the right of' is closer to perception than is 'loves' and has a simpler and less exciting semantics, but its semantics is not that simple either since it has an asymmetrical trajectory-landmark structure (Langacker 1987). When an object, *a*, is said to be to the right of another object, *b*, then object *b* acts as landmark for the trajector a. To capture this property, we placed one object at the centre of the 2-D array whenever the presentation contained a landmark object. This method of placement gave landmark status to the object without the need for separate labels for any of the objects used in the simulation in addition to their different visual appearances and positions. It may be assumed that the concept 'to the right of' is normally learned only by creatures which have independent concepts of the objects perceived in the scene. The setup described circumvents this difficulty without giving way on the crucial issue of systematicity. It might be objected that the system does not learn the completely general concept 'to the right of' but only learns the concept 'to the right of a fixed landmark'. This is true, but we did not consider the objection serious with respect to the principles we wanted to demonstrate. As a matter of fact, our common 'to the right of'—concept is even more complicated than that since it also allows us to change coordinate systems from a viewer-dependent coordinate system to an object-centred co-ordinate system. Again, this does not affect the central point of the demonstration.

The system also had to learn that 'to the right of' is a two-place predicate. When there is only one object in the scene, or when there are more than two objects, the question whether 'this object is to the right of that object (the landmark)' either does not make sense or is ambiguous. In such cases, the system answered 'no' to the question posed to it. On all other presentations one object was placed at the landmark site. A second object was then placed in one of four different positions around the landmark object (right, left, above, or below). We did not teach the network to discriminate among all those positions but simply to respond with a 'yes' if and only if the trajector was positioned to the right of the landmark, and to respond with a 'no' otherwise. In this way, the network was answering the question: 'Is the trajector to the right of the landmark?' If there was no landmark, it responded with a 'no' and if there were three or more objects present, it also responded with a 'no'.

The network was a standard one-layer backpropagation network with graphics facilities for the display of presented objects and running on a PC. The training tolerance for output was 0.1, which means that on a scale from 0 to 1 the network would count 0.9 as correct and stop training when all exemplars in the training set perform above 0.9. The testing tolerance was 0.4 which is sufficient for mechanically distinguishing success and failure. The 2-D picture array measured 8×20 (160 input units). The hidden layer had 30 units and the output layer had 2 units for 'yes' and 'no', respectively. The training set consisted of 6 different objects which were placed in different numbers, positions and combinations and sometimes as landmark, sometimes as trajector. The landmark site and each trajector site consisted of a field of 4 units. The different objects occupied different numbers and combinations of units at a site. The test object set included 3 objects different from the 6 in the training set (see *Figure 1*).

To demonstrate that the network could handle the systematicity of *aRb* and *bRa*, we only trained the network on one of these relations for a given pair of objects while saving the second relation between the pair for the test. Thus, (1) if the network had been trained on '*a* is to the right of *b*', it was not trained on '*b* is to the right of *a*'. In the test phase, the network was shown already familiar objects in combinations it had not encountered before. In addition (2), the network was shown objects it had not encountered before in order to verify that it was able to abstract a sufficiently general concept of '2-D spatial object'. Taken together, (1) and (2) offered sufficient evidence that the network was able to master systematicity from *aRb* to *bRa*; abstraction to the 'right of' concept which we are used to representing as *xRy*; and abstraction over all possible objects in its world, thus successfully taking the set $[a,b,......,i\,]$ as instantiations of *x* and *y* or as legitimate arguments of the relation R.

The training file consisted of 84 training exemplars. The network

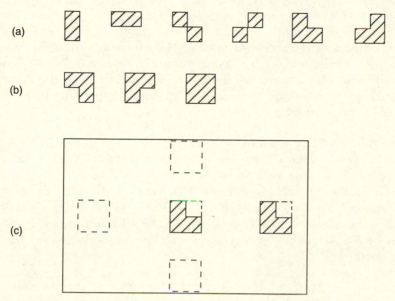

Figure 1. (a) the objects in the training set. (b) the new objects in the test set. (c) an input example.

converged on the desired output in 24 epochs with the mentioned training tolerance of 0.1. The test file consisted of 65 test exemplars. The network was able to generalise successfully within the testing tolerance of 0.4. In other words, systematicity is so simple that a mouse could probably achieve it if its cognitive architecture consists of distributed connectionist networks. It is, therefore, we concluded, no mystery why nature contrives to produce only systematic minds.

5. Objections to System 1

System 1 did not, however, persuade our colleagues that we had fully met F&P's systematicity challenge to distributed connectionism. This section reviews some of their objections.

Objection 1: 'The system is merely a pattern-matcher.' The simplest reply to this objection is: So what? It is not clear why this is an objection as long as the difference between 'mere' pattern-matching and full-fledged systematicity has not been defined. And it is not clear that this distinction has been defined.

Objection 2: 'System 1 does not process semantically complex thoughts.' Here is a simple counter-claim: It does! The trouble is perhaps that we both lack an agreed upon measure of levels of 'semantical complexity' and a clear definition of 'thought' which are not influenced by controversial theoretical prejudice. Intuitively, at least, the thought that something is to the right of something else is not a semantically simple one. This objection leads to the following

Objection 3: 'The system only recognizes *that some 2-D spatial object is to the right of some other 2-D spatial object*. This is not systematicity.' This is an interesting objection because of the need to explain why the representations of System 1 do not exhibit systematicity. The interesting point is that it is far from clear that such an explanation can be provided. Until such an explanation may be forthcoming, let us consider a slightly weakened version of Objection 3:

Objection 4: 'Well, at least it was not the kind of systematicity we had in mind. In fact, the kind of systematicity demonstrated (if any) does not *satisfy the* R(a,b) *requirement. It only satisfies the following, weaker requirement:* Ex & Ey *such that x and y are numerically different spatial objects &* R(x,y). *Basically, your system cannot distinguish between* R(a,b) *and* R(b,a). *It will respond with 'yes' when either of these spatial relations obtain in the scene.'* This is certainly true and to the point. The following reply does not really counter Objection 4: Since System 1 works with real semantic material (objects in visual scenes) it is very probable that its pattern of activation is different when it sees right-of(triangle, square) and right-of(square, triangle).

Objection 4 continued: 'This won't suffice. Here are the crucial points:

(1) Thought at least involves the possibility *of expression of distinctions made, whether in motor behaviour, language or system (or module) output. A difference in patterns of activation is not sufficient for different thoughts to occur.*

(2) Thought requires general concepts. *A dog perceiving a visual scene containing, inter alia, a radio, does not necessarily see (that object as) a radio. Dogs probably lack the concept of a radio, as betrayed by their behaviour.'*

The upshot of this discussion is that systematicity, in some unanticipated sense, may well have been demonstrated by System 1 but that a more complex form of systematicity, one formal expression of which is the relationship between $R(a,b)$ and $R(b,a)$, has yet to be demonstrated by distributed connectionist systems. Just as importantly, however, this will not change the basic structure of the argument of Section 4 above. We already have systematicity and complex thoughts.

6. System 2

The requirements for the new system, System 2, are straightforward in view of what has been said above. The distributed connectionist System 2

- should produce different output for $R(a,b)$ and $R(b,a)$ or, e.g., for right-of(triangle, square) and right-of(square, triangle);
- should necessarily have systematicity; and
- the cognitive mechanisms behind systematicity should be made clear at least to the extent that its necessity has been explained.

For the System 2 simulation a recurrent net was used in order to (1) maintain strict classical syntax in output expression, and (2) fit the hypothesis that thought of a certain complexity may be temporally extended. Point (1) ensures a clean interface between the cognitive module which entertains the thought based on visual perception that, e.g., $R(a,b)$, and a language generation module. Point (2) at least begins to address the topic of the two first objections in Section 5 above. That is, there may actually be differences in complexity between thoughts so that some thoughts need a temporal dimension for their representation whereas other, simpler, thoughts do not. However, this is a hypothesis so far and it is quite possible that ordinary backpropagation networks such as the one used for System 1 might solve the problem addressed by System 2, only using a less clean output syntax. It may be mentioned that a first version of System 2 using recurrent nets and exhibiting the feature of visual attention in order to distinguish between the performance of different cognitive tasks has been described in Bernsen and Ulbaek (1992b). However, the capacity for generalisation of that version was not tested and hence it never demonstrated necessary systematicity.

System 2 is a Tlearn network (due to Jeff Elman, UCSD) running on a SUN. When the network is in recurrent mode there is a copy layer in addition to the hidden layer. The copy layer is used to copy the activity of the hidden layer at time t_1. At time t_2 the activity of the hidden layer at t_1 is fed back into the hidden layer from the copy layer. In this way the network is sensitive to earlier input activity and is able to produce dynamic, temporally discrete output based on static input. System 2 has 100 input units corresponding to a 10 by 10 visual matrix or scene on which 2-D spatial objects of various shapes are shown to it. The hidden layer and the copy layer have 100 units each, and the output layer has six units each one of which, after training, permanently corresponds to one particular named object in the scene. Six different objects, called A, B, C, D, E and F, respectivly, were shown to the system, each occupying part of a 4 by 4 field within the matrix (see *Figure 2*). Six objects allow 30 different right-of orderings between them. Twenty-four of these were used for training and the remaining six orderings were used in the test phase. The six orderings used in the test phase were AB (*'b* is to the right of *a*'), BC, CD, DE, EF and FA. Each static input scene is presented to the network in two consecutive time slices. It is the output which is time-dependent or coded serially. The coding for the presence of, e.g., A anywhere in the scene is:

t_1: 1 0 0 0 0 0
t_2: 0 0 0 0 0 0

Coding for, e.g., A is to the right of B (or BA) is:

t_1: 0 1 0 0 0 0
t_2: 1 0 0 0 0 0

Coding for B is to the right of A (or AB) is:

t_1: 1 0 0 0 0 0
t_2: 0 1 0 0 0 0

In the simulation, no output unit was introduced for expressing the *right of* relation itself. Since the network just recognises one type of spatial relation such an extra output unit is unnecessary, the temporal ordering of the output unit activations performing the distinction between, e.g., *right-of(a,b)* and *right-of(b,a)*. If the network were to be able to recognise more than one kind of spatial relation (e.g., *above(x,y)* as well), units identifying the type of spatial relationship currently attended to would have to be introduced.

System 2 was trained and tested on two successive cognitive tasks. In *Task 1*, the system learns to identify discriminably different individual objects present anywhere in the visual array; e.g., when object *a* is present, the a output unit fires. This way, an *individual object recognition task* is performed requiring the system to develop concepts for each of the spatial objects or object types pre-

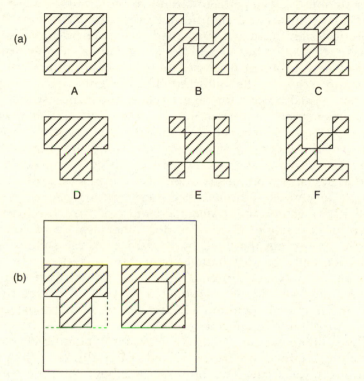

Figure 2. (a) the 2-D objects used. (b) a training input situation in which A is to the right of D.

sented to it. In Task 2, the system learns to identify right-of-ness as obtaining between identified individual objects present any-where in the visual scene. For instance, when *right-of(a,b)* obtains in the visual scene, the output unit representing object b fires before the output unit representing object *a*; when *right-of(b,a)* obtains, the output unit representing object *a* fires before the out-put unit representing object b. This way, a right-of task is learned which is different from, and more complex than that performed by System 1. Subsequently, System 2 was tested on instances of *right-of(x,y)* which it had not encountered during training to verify that the system had succeeded in generalising to the concept *right-of(x,y)* and was able to instantiate to arbitrary combinations of the individual objects known to it.

Recent results from simulations using the version of System 2 described above demonstrate, in my view convincingly, that a dis-tributed connectionist system can solve the systematicity problem posed to System 2. Final work on the simulation will be done in order to obtain a 100 per cent clean test score but does not appear to have any theoretical significance otherwise. The same lack of theoretical significance, it is claimed, would characterise attempts to make the system handle additional semantical complexity to the right-of-ness problem discussed here, of which there are many. The simplest one is the following. The current system knows of 6 different visual objects (or object types) and demonstrates necessary systematicity in its ability to identify right-of-ness with respect to those. There is little doubt that the system, if it were to be taught the identities of new objects, would be able to demonstrate necessary systematicity with respect to those as well. Further semantic complexity abounds even in as simple a concept as *right-of*(x,y) as indicated elsewhere in this paper. System 2 implicitly masters the trajectory-landmark structure described above just as biological systems do. Other aspects of conceptual complexity are not mastered by System 2. These should be handled eventually by distributed connectionist systems, of course, but not as part of a discussion of the systematicity problem. Rather, they should be investigated as part of a research programme in spatial cognition and in the linking of visual and linguistic processing of information.

The training set consisted of the six individual objects and the 24 training right-of orderings located at two thirds of the possible locations in the scene. The input consisted of 1260 time sequences corresponding to 630 different scenes and the network was trained for 2.000.000 epochs. After training the error measure (the total sum of squares) was <0.05. This is hardly sufficient for a 'clean' simulation and explains the remaining errors in the test phase (see below). However, it suffices for the point to be demonstrated here. Nothing was done to make the simulation run quickly and efficiently. The test set consisted of 168 time sequences corresponding to 84 different scenes showing 6 different right-of orderings in two thirds of the possible locations in the scene.

In the test phase, System 2 successfully solved the right-of problem in 57 out of 84 cases if one uses the criterion for success that output from the units corresponding to the observed objects in the proper temporal sequence has to be >0.5 and output from all other units has to be <0.5. This is, however, just one way in which correct results can be mechanically separated from incorrect results. Using the much sharper criterion for success that output from the correct units in correct temporal sequence has to be >0.9 and output from all other units has to be <0.1, System 2 successfully solved the right-of problem in 36 out of 84 cases. However, using an equally mechanically applicable winner-takes-all strategy for success according to which only the two most active output units are selected, System 2 successfully solved the right-of problem in 73 out of 84 cases. Output for the b is to the right of a—problem is shown in Table 1.

a	b	c	d	e	f
0.997	0.018	0.000	0.000	0.000	0.000
0.023	0.997	0.000	0.000	0.000	0.000
0.374	0.030	0.000	0.000	0.000	0.002
0.000	0.546	0.000	0.002	0.000	0.101
0.950	0.006	0.000	0.000	0.000	0.000
0.002	0.998	0.000	0.000	0.000	0.215
0.992	0.422	0.000	0.000	0.000	0.000
0.000	1.000	0.000	0.000	0.000	0.005
1.000	0.002	0.000	0.000	0.000	0.000
0.000	0.969	0.000	0.005	0.111	0.000
0.974	0.000	0.000	0.000	0.000	0.000
0.001	0.999	0.000	0.000	0.000	0.000
0.998	0.000	0.000	0.000	0.000	0.000
0.009	0.627	0.000	0.000	0.000	0.004
0.001	0.998	0.000	0.000	0.000	0.000
0.001	0.947	0.000	0.001	0.002	0.004
0.980	0.003	0.000	0.000	0.000	0.001
0.002	1.000	0.000	0.000	0.000	0.003
1.000	0.022	0.002	0.000	0.000	0.002
0.000	0.994	0.000	0.000	0.003	0.006
0.837	0.000	0.000	0.000	0.000	0.000
0.075	0.638	0.000	0.001	0.072	0.003
1.000	0.000	0.000	0.000	0.000	0.000
0.632	1.000	0.000	0.000	0.000	0.001
0.990	0.016	0.000	0.000	0.000	0.011
0.000	0.995	0.000	0.091	0.000	0.000
1.000	0.000	0.018	0.000	0.000	0.000
0.002	1.000	0.000	0.000	0.000	0.000

Table 1. Test output for System 2 perceiving that b is to the right of a at 14 different scene locations. Two consecutive rows show output corresponding to one static scene

7. Discussion of System 2

It has been established that distributed connectionist nets can learn the following from experience:

- concepts of different 2-D spatial objects or object types (*a, b, c,* etc.) (System 2);
- the concept of 2-D spatial-object(x);
- the concept of right-of(*x,y*) as obtaining between unidentified individual 2-D spatial objects (System 1);
- the concept of right-of(*x,y*) as obtaining between identified individual 2-D spatial objects and, in consequence, the distinction between, e.g., right-of(*a,b*) and right-of(*b,a*) (System 2).

It seems justified to conclude that no further simulation experiments are needed to demonstrate that distributed connectionist nets can exhibit necessary systematicity in the case of a class of two-place asymmetrical predicates. The precise identification of the class of predicates for which distributed connectionist systems are able to exhibit necessary systematicity is not relevant to the systematicity debate.

Moreover, the cognitive mechanisms producing systematicity in System 2 are the same as in System 1. The mechanisms are distributed connectionist versions of abstraction and generalization from experience, and instantiation to experience. It has been known for a long time that distributed connectionist systems are good at performing these conceptual operations.

It is not surprising that System 2 produces necessary systematicity using the very same cognitive mechanisms as does System 1, for the following reason. The spatial input scheme for right-of-ness ($R(a,b)$; $R(a,c)$; $R(c,b)$; etc.) is itself systematic. That is, it involves the same tokens/types, the same spatial relation, and two different types of spatial order due to the asymmetry of the predicate involved. Hence this input scheme can be subjected to the basic cognitive mechanisms of abstraction, generalization and instantiation. It is therefore tempting to propose the general hypothesis that, given a systematic input problem, distributed connectionist systems will necessarily exhibit systematicity. Only the complexity, in some sense to be discovered, of some class of systematicity problems may limit the scope of the hypothesis just stated. However, this complexity issue is only accidentally related to the systematicity problem discussed here.

Given the performance of System 2, it appears highly likely that a system of this kind might exhibit necessary inferential systematicity (cf. Section 2 above). Inferential systematicity would be found in a system which, necessarily, if it were able to conclude *a* from, e.g., *a&b* and *a&b&c&d&e*, would also be able to conclude *a* from, e.g., *a&b&c* (F&P 1988). What a system with inferential systematicity has to learn is, e.g., an abstract schema for propositional inference from conjunctions. The abstraction is the following. It does not matter how many conjuncts (or members) you have in a set or which they are: you are always allowed to infer a subset of the conjuncts from the set. We have already seen the general character of the distributed connectionist mechanisms needed for this cognitive task.

It would appear that the systematicity problem has been solved to the advantage of distributed connectionism. However, there is a final twist to the issue which will be addressed in the next section.

8. Mere Implementation?

If distributed connectionist systems produce necessary systematicity, there seems to be only line of objection left for maintaining that the classical symbolic paradigm is the only general computational paradigm for cognitive science. This line of objection is to claim that the demonstration provided above, just like all other purported demonstrations of systematicity in connectionism to date, is just another demonstration that distributed connectionism may implement classical cognitive architectures (cf. the assumption made in Section 3 above). In other words, despite all that has been said so far, Systems 1 and 2 merely implement classical syntax and that is why they demonstrate necessary systematicity.

On the face of it, this claim may appear quite unreasonable. So far, we have had no reason whatsoever to believe that distributed connectionist systems have classical syntax. On the contrary, their difference from classical systems is precisely that they do not have classical syntax. They take the same (systematic) input material as do classical systems and they have the same (systematic and, by design, syntactic) output performance as have classical systems. But what happens in between input and output is done by processing algorithms that are profoundly different from classical algorithms. Moreover, the entire explanation provided above of why distributed systems produce necessary systematicity has been offered at *the cognitive level via* conceptual operations such as abstraction, generalization and instantiation scoping concepts and relations. So, again, the objection we are now considering would appear preposterous. Why is this objection still to be anticipated, all appearance to the contrary notwithstanding? In attempting to answer this question, I shall distinguish between three different issues. Once this has been done, it may have become clear why the burden of proof is now on the classicalists if the systematicity issue is to be kept alive.

1. Information processed and the processing of that information: The question whether distributed connectionist systems merely implement classical syntax is, in fact, ambiguous. The ambiguity lies in the *task (or input) domains* addressed by those systems. Here are the possibilities. We may be dealing with either:

(a) distributed connectionist systems working within the task domain of explicit symbols and classical syntax, possibly modified by the addition of statistical linguistic material in accordance with current trends in computational linguistics. One example among many is the parallel distributed processing of a combination of hard symbolic and syntactic rules and soft symbolic linguistic rules which incorporate corpus-derived numerical values. Of course, even in this case adherents of distributed connectionism maintain that no classical syntax is involved in the actual processing of input domain information. Such distributed connectionist systems may realize a universal Turing (LISP) machine which has no complexity boundary to its computations whatsoever (e.g., Smolensky *et al.* 1992);

or with

(b) distributed connectionist systems working within task domains that contain no explicit symbols and no explicit syntax. The example at hand is the parallel distributed processing of 'real' semantic information (i.e., visual representations) done by Systems 1 and 2 above. Again it is claimed that no classical syntax is involved in the actual processing of input domain information. Of course, the input information is itself systematic (cf. above), but that is an obvious requirement for the systems to be able to address the systematicity problem in the first place.

The relevant difference between cases (a) and (b) is the following: In (a), symbolic and syntactic information is *literally being processed* albeit in a distributed connectionist manner. This information is out there in the input. It is therefore not surprising if Smolensky et al. are still in for the criticism that they merely implement classical syntax. They are actually close to admitting as much themselves (Smolensky *et al.* 1992). In (b), on the other hand, there is no explicit symbolic information (rules or symbolic representations) anywhere, except in the output. In this case, symbolic and syntactic information is not literally being processed. It does not make sense to speak of 'mere implementation' here because we have an explanation at the right, i.e., cognitive level involving concepts, relations, order, abstraction, generalisation and instantiation. So the ambiguity mentioned is one between two completely different issues: (1) *what* (input) information is literally being processed? (2) how is the information being processed?

It is not the task of the present author to advise Smolensky and other distributed connectionists on anything. But it does seem odd, if not downright absurd, if the purportedly fundamental problem of systematicity can be solved, for certain classes of input domains, at least, such as the literal processing of symbolic and syntactic information, by merely looking at the task or input domain addressed by a distributed connectionist system, as fol- lows: Is your distributed system processing explicit linguistic information? 'Yes.' But then your system is a mere implementa- tion of a classical architecture! Some may still want to pursue this line of argument against one class of distributed connectionist sim- ulations purporting to demonstrate systematicity but that will not be done here. In any case, such a strategy of argument would not be a general one because there are important classes of input domains relevant to the systematicity problem which do not involve explicit linguistic information, such as those of the Systems 1 and 2 above. The two remaining issues to be dealt with in this section address the general case.

2. The cognitive level and the algorithmic level: The story to be told about System 2 at the cognitive level goes as follows. System 2 learns the concepts of individual objects (or object types) which can enter into the spatial relation right-of. This way, System 2 is well under way to acquiring a general concept of 2-D spatial object(x) as denoting the kind of entities which may enter into this relationship. Furthermore, System 2 learns the general concept of the ordered relation right-of(x,y) in such a way that, given two individual 2-D spatial objects (or object types) known to it, it is capable of deciding which object is to the right of which other individual object. I see no reason why classicalists and distributed connectionists might not agree on this story about how any cogni- tive system identifies a right-of relationship between two different spatial objects known to it. They may disagree on the nature of the concepts and relations involved, but that is a different matter to be considered below.

At the *algorithmic level*, however, System 2 involves no classical syntax and no classical constituents since the algorithms work at the level of individual processing units in a distributed system of representation. When System 2 perceives *aRb* and outputs correctly, it must clearly activate its representations of *a*, *b* and *right-of-ness* and create the correct representation *aRb*. Given the distributed nature of its processing of information, there is every reason to assume that what happens is not that the representations of *a* and *b* are separately activated and, as such, with no further changes to their activation patterns enter into a relation with an equally separately activated representation of *right-of-ness*. Distributed connectionist systems do not work that way since they do not have classical constituents, but classical systems do. Similarly, when System 2 perceives *bRa* and outputs correctly, it must activate its representations of *a*, *b* and *right-of-ness* and create the correct representation *bRa*. It is possible that more or less the same set of units become active in this case as in the case of *aRb*, but the resulting vector which determines the output has to be different in the two cases.

3. Implicit and explicit internal systematicity: If this is still not the way to solve the systematicity problem, we are back to the intriguing possibility that System 2 above is a mere implementation of a classical and syntactical cognitive architecture. How could this be decided? The point is that *we don't have a clue*. We do not have the faintest idea of how, by looking into the way that System 2 processes information, we were to decide that, all appearances to the contrary notwithstanding, System 2 is nevertheless a mere implementation of a classical architecture (Brian McLaughlin has admitted as much in personal communication. This admission may be temporary, of course.).

So here are the options: We either deem the systematicity problem solved along the lines indicated or we wait until we get a clue as to how it may be decided whether, e.g., System 2 really is an implementation of a classical cognitive architecture. *If* such a clue or, rather, set of criteria, come forward; *if* they are operational (i.e., intersubjectively applicable to real systems); and *if* by using them it turns out that System 2 is an implementation of a classical architecture, then the current author would have to confess to being a classicalist after all. Meanwhile, there are good reasons to conclude that the existence proof of just one distributed connectionist system, whatever be its input domain, which is able to exhibit necessary systematicity is all it takes to refute the classicalist position. For the same good reasons, if, at the end of the day, this turns out not to be true, it is quite possible that the classicalist position will have become so rarefied in the process of further development that nobody would object to it.

Let us look at the foothold, as it were, of the classicalist scenario just outlined. It is that connectionism will have solved the systematicity issue only when it has provided a so far missing level of account of distributed processing of information:

> ...[connectionism must] explain the existence of [systematicity] without assuming that mental processes are causally sensitive to the constituent structure of mental representations. (Fodor and McLaughlin 1990)

It is not clear why connectionism should accept this challenge. Otherwise, the classicalist position runs the risk of becoming, once again, trivially true, which it certainly is not, given its conception of constituent structure. The story told above clearly does assume that the mental processes generating systematicity are causally sensitive to the constituent structure of mental representations. Consider the following simple argument: Systematicity in both the input and the output requires systematicity in between. If this argument is true, then there's got to be causal sensitivity in distributed connectionist systems to the constituent structure of mental representations (i.e., of concepts, relations, order, predicates, etc.). System 2 above, for instance, satisfies the condition that there is systematicity in both the input and the output even though its task domain is not linguistic.

It may now be pointed out that a look-up table, for instance, might satisfy the condition that there is systematicity in both the input and the output. However, the *internal* systematicity in between might be said to be at most *implicit*; it is not *explicit* as in classical systems. System 2 is not a look-up table. This is proved by its capacities for generalization and generation. The (fortunate) fact that System 2 is not merely a look-up table can hardly by itself constitute a proof of the classicalist position. However, from this fact one might go on to conjecture that if the internal systematicity in between input and output in distributed connectionist systems is explicit rather than implicit, then such systems are implementations of classical architectures after all. It follows that as long as it is not known whether distributed systems have explicit internal systematicity or not, connectionism has not answered the systematicity challenge:

> We still don't have a substantive [constituent level] connectionist account of systematicity. (Fodor and McLaughlin 1990)

Instead of using the term 'explicit internal systematicity', Fodor and McLaughlin point out that, on the classicalist view, the representations *aRb* and *bRa* literally have the same parts and call this 'real constituency'. Does System 2 have real constituency? If the criterion for real constituency is that System 2 does represent, in both cases, and at the cognitive level, the external objects a and b and the relation R between them, then the answer is clearly affirmative. If the criterion is the syntactic symbol system hypothesis, then the answer would *seem* to be just as clearly negative: both System 1 and System 2 just behave as if they know of classical syntax but they don't know of classical syntax. The very same units, more or less, may be active in both the aRb and bRa cases, but so far this has not been stated as a criterion for satisfying the classicalist position. If exactly the same units are active in the two cases, should they be equally active? Or should they be equally active within a certain margin of tolerance? Which margin? Why? If not exactly the same units are active in both cases, which is possible and even likely, then what? Are there principled margins of tolerance to be observed? Why? In other words, we simply don't know what 'real constituency' means in distributed connectionist terms. The same argument *seems* to apply to the question whether System 2 has 'combinatorial constituent structure'. It has—at the cognitive level. At the algorithmic level we have no idea of what that might mean in distributed connectionist terms.

Finally, the claim *seems* clearly justified that the structure of the complex representation which System 2 has (e.g., aRb or bRa) has a causal role in the generation of its behaviour: the system responds systematically differently depending on which one of these complex representations it has. In F&P's terminology (1988), when the system's representations of a, b, and R are simultaneously active and the system has the complex representation aRb, then we also have to admit that the system's representations of a, b, and R enter into a specific kind of 'construction' with each other. This construction differs from the construction among a, b, and R when the system has the complex representation bRa. So, the constituency relations are themselves semantically significant at the cognitive level as F&P claim they should be. At the algorithmic level, however, we do not know what the kind of 'construction' required is.

In summary, then, and combining the cognitive and algorithmic levels descriptions, the distributed connectionist representation *a is to the right of b* therefore seems to be a *non*-atomic mental representation having *non*-syntactic structure. It therefore *seems* to be just false to maintain that

> ... we cannot have both a combinatorial representational system and a connectionist architecture at the cognitive level.

The classicalist position seems confused because the cognitive and algorithmic levels are not kept distinct in the systematicity argument. Once they are kept distinct, it becomes obvious that what is so far an uncontroversial cognitive level story is being combined with an algorithmic level story to which there exists an equally valid alternative.

It is true that things are not always what they seem. The trouble is, however, that we don't know what to look for in order to decide whether, e.g., System 2 is after all an implementation of a classical architecture. We don't have a clue as to what constitutes a generic concept of 'explicit internal systematicity' such that:

(1) this concept might subsume not only well-known instances of classical syntactic processing of information but also instances of distributed connectionist processing of information characterized by systematicity; and

(2) if this concept were applicable to distributed connectionist systems exhibiting necessary systematicity then these would count as implementations of classical architectures rather than alternatives to them.

Classicalist might want to argue that this concept of explicit internal systematicity is not generic at all: it is simply the classical concept of constituent structure. But this simply won't do. As demonstrated, we have no idea as to how the concept of explicit internal systematicity should be applied to the algorithmic processing of systematic distributed connectionist systems in order to determine whether they implement classical syntax or constituent structure or not. The classicalist position has so far not been geared to answer this question and it is perhaps not likely that it will be able to do so.

9. Conclusion

Several times above I have mentioned the agreement between classicalists and distributed connectionists about what takes place at the cognitive level of description in systems mastering systematicity. There are limits to this agreement, however, and this may turn out to have important implications for the *algorithmic* analysis of systems handling systematicity in 'real' semantic domains. It should not be forgotten that classicalists and distributed connectionists tend to disagree on what are the 'constituents' of thought. This problem *is* a substantial unsolved problem of cognitive science as witnessed by the fact that even within the core domain of the classicalist position, i.e., that of linguistic syntax, it is becoming increasingly clear that expert syntacticians disagree profoundly and perhaps incurably about the correct parsing of ordinary sentences. If the constitutents of thought are to a considerable extent non-classical, i.e., irreducible to the scheme of rules and (atomic and molecular) representations and their tokenings as causal syntactic entities, as distributed connectionists maintain, this would provide substantial evidence against the classicalist algorithmic story of what goes on in systems mastering systematicity and therefore against the classicalist position as a whole.

The conclusion reached in Section 7 above would therefore seem to stand up for the time being. Some might want to take this opportunity to leave the increasingly thin philosophical air zone of the systematicity problem and do more substantial cognitive science instead. Cognitive science still needs to provide an acceptable account of concepts, relations and predicates at both the cognitive, algorithmic and implementational levels. It is a qualified guess that this account will incorporate aspects which have been stressed by classicalists as well as aspects which have been stressed by distributed connectionists. Obviously, the demonstration that distributed connectionist systems can exhibit necessary systematicity in a way different from classical systems does not, by itself, give distributed connectionist cognitive architectures any advantage over classical architectures.

References

Ajjanagadde, V. and Shastri, L. 1991. 'Rules and variables in neural nets', *Neural Computation* **3**, 121–134.

Bernsen, N. O. and Ulbæk, I. 1992a. 'Two games in town. Systematicity in distributed connectionist systems', *Artificial Intelligence and Simulation of Behaviour Quarterly*, Special Issue on Hybrid Models of Cognition Part 2, No. 79, 25–30.

Bernsen, N. O. and Ulbæk, I. 1992b. 'Systematicity, thought and attention in a distributed connectionist system', *Working Papers in Cognitive Science* WPCS-92-2, Centre of Cognitive Science, Roskilde University.

Bernsen, N. O. and Kopp, L. 1993. 'A connectionist architecture for spatial cognition' (in preparation).

Fodor, J. A. and McLaughlin, B. P. 1990. 'Connectionism and the problem of systematicity: Why Smolensky's solution doesn't work', *Cognition* **35**, 183–204.

Fodor, J. A. and Pylyshyn, Z. W. 1988. 'Connectionism and cognitive architecture: A Critical Analysis', *Cognition* **28**, 3–71.

Langacker, R. W. 1987. *Foundations of Cognitive Grammar*. Stanford CA: Stanford University Press.

Pylyshyn, Z. W. 1984. *Computation and Cognition: Toward a Foundation for Cognitive Science*. Cambridge MA: MIT Press.

Smolensky, P. 1987. 'The constituent structure of connectionist mental states: A reply to Fodor and Pylyshyn', *Southern Journal of Philosophy* **26**, Supplement, 137–161.

Smolensky, P. 1988. 'On the proper treatment of connectionism', *Behavioral and Brain Sciences* **11**, 1–74.

Smolensky, P., Legendre, G. and Miyata, Y. 1992. 'Principles for an integrated connectionist/symbolic theory of higher cognition', *Report* 92-08, Institute for Cognitive Science, University of Colorado at Boulder.

Systematicity, Conceptual Truth, and Evolution*

BRIAN P. McLAUGHLIN

1. The Fodor–Pylyshyn Challenge to Connectionists

In their seminal 1988 paper, 'Connectionism and cognitive architecture', Fodor and Pylyshyn posed a challenge to connectionists: to say how connectionism could explain systematic relationships among cognitive capacities without implementing a classical cognitive architecture. Unless this challenge can be met, they argued, connectionists will not have told us how connectionism can provide an *adequate alternative* theory of cognition to the classical theory of cognition. For if connectionism fails to explain systematic relationships among cognitive capacities ('systematicity', for short) then it will fail to be an adequate theory of cognition. And if connectionism explains systematicity by implementing a classical cognitive architecture, then connectionism will fail to be an alternative theory of cognition to the classical one.

2. Types of Responses to the Challenge

The systematicity challenge has invoked a flood of responses. Subtleties aside, the respondents fall into two broad camps. One camp attempts to meet the challenge: members of this camp attempt to say how connectionism could explain systematicity without implementing a classical cognitive architecture.[1] The second camp declines the challenge, claiming that it need not be met. The members of this camp deny Fodor's and Pylyshyn's implied condition of adequacy for a cognitive theory, namely that an adequate cognitive theory must explain systematicity. If members of this camp are correct, then, of course, connectionists need not meet the Fodor–Pylyshyn challenge; for an adequate cognitive theory need not explain systematicity.

* I wish to thank Andrew Gleeson, Ackim Stephen, and Fritz Warfield for many helpful discussions of issues addressed here. Sections 4 and 5 of this paper overlap quite extensively with section 5 of McLaughlin (1993b). I thank Kluwer for permission to use the material in question from McLaughlin (1993).
[1] See, e.g., Smolensky (1991).

This second camp divides into three subcamps, which I will now characterize in a rough and ready way, without pausing for qualifications. One subcamp denies the adequacy condition on the grounds that it is not the case that there are systematic relationships among cognitive capacities.[2] The two remaining subcamps, in contrast, at least purport to concede that there are systematically related cognitive capacities. But one subcamp claims that systematic relationships among cognitive capacities hold as a matter of conceptual necessity, and for this reason denies that systematicity is a phenomenon to be explained by an empirical theory.[3] The other subcamp concedes that systematicity requires an empirical explanation, but denies that a theory of cognition must yield such an explanation. This subcamp maintains that systematic relationships among cognitive capacities can be explained by evolutionary biology, rather than by a theory of cognition. Evolutionary biology can, this subcamp maintains, explain systematicity in terms of natural selection. The leading idea is that systematically related cognitive capacities are co-adaptive, and, as a result, were selected for.[4]

3. What Lies Ahead

In what follows, I will focus exclusively on these last two subcamps of the camp that denies the adequacy condition. I will thus say nothing about attempts to show how connectionism could explain systematicity without implementing a classical cognitive architecture.[5] And I will not attempt to argue that there are systematically related cognitive capacities.[6] My primary aim here is modest: to explain Fodor's and Pylyshyn's adequacy condition for a theory of cognition and to respond to some leading attempts to deny it.

I will proceed as follows. I will first say what systematicity is. I will then say how classicism proposes to explain it. After that, I will turn to respondents who deny the adequacy condition.

---

[2] This appears to be Dennett's position (Dennett 1991).

[3] See, e.g., Clark (1988; 1989; 1991).

[4] See Braddon-Mitchell & Fitzpatrick (1990); and Sterelny (1990).

[5] For a response to Paul Smolensky's attempts to do so, see McLaughlin (1987) and Fodor and McLaughlin (1990). For a discussion of some of the other leading attempts to meet the challenge, see McLaughlin (1993b).

[6] Nor will I discuss the allures of connectionism as an alternative to the classical theory of cognition. For such a discussion, see McLaughlin and Warfield (forthcoming).

4. What is Systematicity?

The answer to this question has not, I believe, been made sufficiently clear by classicists.[7] As a result, there have been some misunderstandings of what systematicity is. I won't attempt to sort
through all the misunderstandings. Instead, I will spell out the
core phenomenon of cognitive systematicity in detail.

To begin, cognitive capacities are not fundamental capacities:
possession of a cognitive capacity consists in possession of other
capacities. Cognitive capacities thus have what we will call 'constitutive bases': there are other capacities possession of which constitutes possession of the capacities in question. A theory of cognition
should explain what possession of cognitive capacities consists in;
it should describe constitutive bases for such capacities. Thus, to
use a phrase of Cummins's (Cummins 1983), a theory of cognition
should provide 'functional analyses' of cognitive capacities. As we
will see shortly, systematic relationships between cognitive capacities impose a condition of adequacy on any functional analyses of
the capacities in question.

Consider the following four pairs of cognitive capacities:

(1) the capacity to believe that the dog is chasing the cat *and* the
capacity to believe that the cat is chasing the dog,
(2) the capacity to think that if the cat runs, then the dog will *and*
the capacity to think that if the dog runs, then the cat will,
(3) the capacity to see a visual stimulus as a square above a triangle
and the capacity to see a visual stimulus as a triangle above a
square, and
(4) the capacity to prefer a green triangular object to a red square
object *and* the capacity to prefer a red triangular object to a
green square object.

Notice that the two members of each pair are alike in the following
two ways:

(I) they are capacities to have intentional states in the same
intentional mode (e.g., preference, belief, seeing as), and
(II) the intentional states in question have related contents.

(I) should be clear enough. To comment briefly on (II), the contents
of the members of a pair are, of course, distinct; and neither content
implies the other. None the less, the contents are related. Notice that

---

[7] Matthews (1991) and Sterelny (1990) have complained about this, not
without justification.

we use the same words to specify each. For now, we can take whether or not we use the same words to specify each content as a fairly reliable operational test for whether or not two types of intentional states have contents that are related in the sense intended in (II).

There is an astronomical number of pairs of cognitive capacities whose two members are related in ways (I) and (II).[8] For example, when R is not an asymmetrical relationship, there will be an astronomical number of pairs of cognitive capacities whose members are of the forms, respectively, the capacity to think that a R b (e.g., the dog is chasing the cat) and the capacity to think that b R a (e.g., the cat is chasing the dog). Moreover, a *typical* possessor of one member of a pair *would* possess the other member as well; that is, except in exceptional cases that call for special explanation, a possessor of one member would have the other too.[9]

According to classicists, the reason that there are the sorts of counterfactual dependencies in question is that capacities alike in ways (I) and (II) are 'intrinsically connected', rather than 'punctate'.[10] Pairs of capacities alike in ways (I) and (II) are 'intrinsically connected' in they have connected constitutive bases, rather than discrete constitutive bases; and thus they are not 'punctate' capacities with respect to each other. The exercises of the capacities in question are operations of an underlying *system* of elements and operations.

Here is what it is for two capacities (of any sort whatsoever) to be systematically related: two capacities are systematically related if and only if they have constitutive bases such that a typical possessor of the one capacity would possess the other. According to classicists, capacities alike in ways (I) and (II) are systematically related in that sense.

Systematic relationships between the members of pairs of capacities alike in ways (I) and (II) impose a condition of adequacy on any would-be functional analyses of the capacities in question: that the analyses describe constitutive bases for the members of such relevant pairs of capacities that will yield an explanation of why a typical possessor of one member of a pair would possess the other. And this condition of adequacy on functional analyses of the capacities in question yields a condition of adequacy on a theory of cognition: that it offer functional analyses that meet this condition of

[8] It should be mentioned that a particular capacity will often be pairwise related in ways (I) and (II) to a number of capacities. There are families of capacities whose members are pairwise related in ways (I) and (II).

[9] Exceptional cases will include, for example, certain kinds of aphasia.

[10] This terminology is Fodor's and Pylyshyn's (see Fodor and Pylyshyn 1988).

adequacy. By 'cognitive systematicity', or 'systematicity', for short, let us mean systematic relationships between the members of pairs of capacities related in ways (I) and (II).[11] A theory will, then, be able to explain systematicity if and only if it offers functional analyses that meet the condition of adequacy in question. The functional analyses of the members of a pair of capacities alike in ways (I) and (II) should thus yield explanations of the following counterfactual dependency relationship they bear to each other: that a typical possessor of one would possess the other.

Classicists maintain that the members of a relevant pair of capacities can be functionally analysed into *common* capacities and (second-order) capacities for their joint exercise. These capacities *constitute* possession of the members of pairs of capacities alike in ways (I) and (II).[12] And it is because of this 'intrinsic connection', to use Fodor's and Pylyshyn's phrase, between the capacities that a typical possessor of one member of such a pair would have the other.

5. How Classicism Proposes to Explain Systematicity

On the classical view of cognition, the two members of any of pairs (1)–(4), for example, will have constitutive bases that involve possession of the same concepts, a capacity or faculty for jointly exercising the concepts in either of the two ways appropriate to the contents of the two relevant intentional states, and a capacity to token intentional states in the intentional mode in question (e.g., preference, belief, seeing-as, etc.).[13] For example, there are bases for the capacity to believe that *the dog is chasing the cat* and the capacity to believe that *the cat is chasing the dog* that involve

---

[11] This is a somewhat narrower notion of systematicity than the one Fodor and Pylyshyn (1988) used. If we expand (I) to include intentional acts (and so, for example, speech acts) and intentional activities (e.g., inferring), in addition to intentional states, then the notions will, I believe, be equivalent.

[12] A terminological point: for stylistic variety, I will, hereafter, sometimes refer to pairs of capacities related in ways (I) and (II) as 'relevant pairs of capacities'.

[13] It may be denied that seeing-as involves the exercise of concepts. I would argue that it does: to see something as (say) a cat is to exercise the concept of a cat. However, seeing-as also involves visual percepts, and visual percepts are distinct from concepts (see, e.g., Dretske 1978, McLaughlin 1989, Crane 1992b, Peacocke 1992, and Tye 1992). (See footnote 15.)

(a) the same concepts (the concept of a dog, the concept of a cat, the concept of chasing),

(b) a capacity for jointly exercising the concepts in a way appropriate to having intentional states with the contents in question (the content that the dog is chasing the cat and the content that the cat is chasing the dog), and

(c) a capacity to have an intentional state in the intentional mode in question (belief).

The contents of the intentional states in question are related in that they involve the exercise of essentially the same concepts. The contents are different because of differences in the specific way the concepts are jointly exercised. And of course both capacities involve the capacity to have beliefs. Given that the bases of the capacity to believe that the dog is chasing the cat and the capacity to believe that the cat is chasing the dog include (a)–(c), we can readily see why a typical possessor of the one capacity would possess the other.

Now classicism offers specific proposals concerning what possession of concepts consists in, concerning how concepts are jointly exercised, and concerning what the various intentional modes consist in. But before turning to those proposals, some background in is order. To begin, classicism postulates a cognitive architecture which includes a system of mental symbols (or mental representations) with a compositional syntax.[14] It is because a classical cognitive architecture possesses this feature that it is referred to as a 'language of thought architecture' (Fodor 1975).[15] Moreover, a classical architecture includes a system of types of algorithmic processes. The processes are types of symbolic processes: they consist of types of causal transitions from symbols to symbols, where symbols are typed by their formal, rather than their semantic, properties. Symbols par-

---

[14] It is widely claimed by classicists that the system of mental representation will also have a compositional semantics. But whether that is so is an empirical issue. It is not an *essential* feature of a classical cognitive architecture that it include a system of mental representation with a compositional semantics, though it is essential that it include a system with a compositional syntax. (See Schiffer 1991.)

[15] It should be noted that classicism is not committed to the view that all mental symbols (or representations) are linguistic (see Fodor 1982, McLaughlin 1987; 1989). Classicism can allow, for example, that some mental symbols are 'imagistic' rather than linguistic. What classicism is committed to is that symbols function as linguistic symbols when they are constituents of thoughts, i.e., propositional attitudes. It is, however, consistent with classicism, as I understand it, that there are what Goldman (1986) calls 'sense-linked' mental codes. As I indicated earlier, I think that there are percepts (visual, auditory, etc.); and percepts are

ticipate in such causal processes in virtue of their formal properties, but not in virtue of their semantic properties. However, even though symbols do not participate in the processes in virtue of their semantic properties, the processes will be such that the symbol transitions make sense, given the meanings of the symbols. These causal processes will thus satisfy criteria of semantic coherence. It is because of this feature that the classical conception of cognition is often referred to as 'the proof-theoretic conception'.

Classicism proposes to explain the various intentional modes that are the various 'propositional attitudes' (belief, desire, etc.) by appeal to different computational relations that an organism can bear to a mental symbol with a propositional content. The content of such an intentional state is just the meaning or content of the mental symbol in question.[16] So, for example, on the classical view, believing that P consists in bearing a computational relation constitutive of belief to a mental symbol that means that P.[17] Concepts are understood to be capacities to token certain sorts of mental symbols with 'incomplete contents' as constituents of symbols with propositional or 'complete' contents; the former are mental 'words', the latter are mental 'sentences'. Concepts are thus capacities to token mental

---

[16] It is the task of a psychosemantic theory to tell us what content primitive mental symbols have. A psychosemantic theory *must*, I believe, take into account noncomputational factors, indeed even factors that are external to the cognizer. A purely computational account of content is thus simply not to be had, though content *may* prove to have a narrow functional component (see McLaughlin 1993a). But, having noted that, I will not discuss here the form a psychosemantic theory might take. Suffice it to note that without the aid of a psychosemantic theory, neither classicism nor connectionism will succeed in providing functional analyses of capacities to have intentional states. (For two different psychosemantic theories that are both *consistent* with the classical account of cognitive architecture, see Fodor (1990) and Dretske (1991).)

[17] Here I oversimplify. There is very likely no single computational relation constitutive of belief, or of desire, or of the like. 'Belief' and 'desire', for instance, are blanket terms that cover a wide range of different intentional modes. For example , 'belief' covers deeply held convictions as well as superficial options; 'desire' covers thought out preferences as well as momentary urges.

---

not concepts, and not mental words. I lack the space here to discuss intentional states (e.g., visual experiences) that do not contain concepts as constituents; a proper discussion must await another occasion. But I wish to note for the record that there are systematically related capacities to have such intentional states, and that explaining those systematic relationships without implementing a classical architecture with sense-linked symbols is a formidable challenge to connectionism.

'words' in mental 'sentences'. The content of a concept will be the content of the mental word in question.

Here, then, is how classicism proposes to explain systematic relations among capacities such as (1)–(4). The capacities will, according to classicism, have constitutive bases that include the capacity to token the same mental words, a faculty for constructing out of the words mental sentences that have the same contents as the contents of either of the two relevant intentional states, and the capacity to undergo computational processes with either of the mental sentences in question in a way constitutive of the relevant intentional mode. Thus, classicism postulates constitutive bases for pairs of capacities such as (1)–(4) which explain why a typical possessor of one member of such a pair would have the other too.

The challenge Fodor and Pylyshyn pose to connectionists is, you will recall, to say how connectionism could explain systematicity without implementing a classical cognitive architecture. To explain systematicity, connectionists must postulate constitutive bases for capacities alike in ways (I) and (II) that are such that, given that the capacities have those constitutive bases, a typical possessor of one of the capacities would possess the other.

Connectionists typically invoke concepts in their accounts of intentional states.[18] And it is open to a connectionist to maintain, for example, that the capacities to believe *that the dog is chasing the cat* and to believe *that the cat is chasing the dog* have constitutive bases which include (a)–(c). But connectionists should, then, tell us how connectionism could provide a computational account of concepts and capacities for their joint exercise that is different from the classical account. That these capacities to have intentional states involve the possession of concepts and a faculty for their joint exercise does not, of course, *logically* imply that individuals who have the capacities have a classical cognitive architecture. Classicism offers a bold empirical hypothesis concerning what possession of a concept consists in, and concerning how capacities are jointly exercised. Connectionists who postulate concepts and capacities for their joint exercise owe us a sketch of an alternative to the classical account of such matters; and, it should go without saying, the alternative should not be one we already know is false. Now connectionists might eschew postulation of concepts and capacities for their joint exercise. But if they do, then they should tell us how they propose to explain systematic relationships between pairs of capacities such as (1)–(4) without

---

[18] See, for example, Rumelhart and McClelland (1986).

invoking concepts and capacities for their joint exercise. In sum, then, in order to meet the Fodor–Pylyshyn challenge for capacities of the sort cited in (1)–(4), connectionists must at least either (A) tell us how connectionism could offer an account of concepts and of capacities for their joint exercise which does not imply the classical account, or else (B) tell us how connectionism could explain systematic relationships between the members of such pairs of capacities without invoking concepts and capacities for their joint exercise.

So far, connectionists have not met the challenge; and I think that their prospects for doing so are truly dim.[19] But as I noted earlier, I will be concerned here not with attempts to meet the challenge, but rather with attempts to show that the challenge need not be met. More specifically, I will focus on attempts to show that the challenge need not be met which none the less concede that capacities alike in ways (I) and (II) are such that a typical possessor of one would possess the other, and which also concede that:

(CA) a condition of adequacy on a cognitive theory is that it provide functional analyses of capacities to have intentional states.

Anyone who rejects (CA) will, of course, reject the claim that it is a condition of adequacy on a cognitive theory that it explain systematicity. I will have nothing to say here to connectionists who reject (CA), beyond this: if connectionism does not seek to tell us what possession of capacities to have intentional states consists in, then connectionism and classicism are not in competition. Classicism proposes to offer functional analysis of capacities to have intentional states. And the explanation of systematicity is a condition of adequacy on theories that purport to offer functional analyses of such capacities. If connectionism does not purport to offer such functional analyses, then the issue of explaining systematicity does not arise for connectionism. But if connectionism does not purport to offer such analyses, then it does not purport to offer an alternative theory of intentional phenomena to the classical theory. To repeat: connectionism and classicism would not, then, be in competition.

In what remains, I will focus exclusively on attempts to show that while (CA) is true and there are counterfactual dependencies between capacities alike in ways (I) and (II), it is not a condition of adequacy on a cognitive theory that it explain systematicity.

[19] See McLaughlin (1993b).

6. Is it Conceptually True that Cognition is Systematic ?

The claim that capacities to have intentional states are systematically related implies that if C and C* are capacities that are alike in ways (I) and (II), then

(CG) A typical possessor of C would have C*.

Hereafter, when I speak of counterfactuals of type (CG), I will mean generalizations of form (CG) that are such that the C and C* they cite are capacities alike in ways (I) and (II), that is, capacities to have intentional states in the same intentional mode and with related contents. I want now to turn to the epistemic status of counterfactual generalizations of type (CG).

Andy Clark (1991) tells us that: 'The systematicity of thoughts, as ascribed using ordinary sentences, is a conceptual requirement if we are to be justified in finding any thoughts at all' (p. 205). It is, Clark maintains, a conceptual truth that certain thoughts are, 'ceteris paribus', systematically related. If I understand him, by this he means that when two capacities are alike in ways (I) and (II), it will be a conceptual truth that, ceteris paribus, a possessor of one such capacity would possess the other.[20] Clark thus does not commit himself to the view that possession of one member of a pair is logically necessary and sufficient for possession of the other. His idea seems to be, rather that possession of one member of a pair is, as a matter of conceptual necessity, a (defeasible) a priori criterion for possession of the other. Put in our terms, Clark (1991) seems to hold that counterfactual generalizations of type (CG) are conceptual truths, rather than 'contingent, empirical' truths (p. 202), as Fodor and Pylyshyn hold.[21]

The issue of whether counterfactual generalizations of type (CG) are 'contingent' truths or 'conceptual' truths is a complex one. I lack the space to address it properly here. I will, then, for the sake of argument and brevity, concede for the nonce Clark's point that counterfactual generalizations of type (CG) are conceptual truths. Let us see how the Fodor-Pylyshyn challenge to connectionists fares if this is true.

Clark tells us that in taking it to be an empirical truth that 'cognition is systematic', Fodor and Pylyshyn 'misconceive the *nature*

---

[20] See also Clark (1988; 1989).

[21] Clark cites Gareth Evan's (Evans, 1982) 'generality constraint' in support of this. In a lucid and instructive paper, Martin Davies (1991) very nicely develops Evan's 'generality constraint' argument, underscoring its connection with systemacity.

of thought-ascription, and with it the significance of systematicity'
(p. 201). Clark (1991) goes on to say that

> (i) What stands in need of empirical explanation is not the sys-
> tematicity of *thoughts* but (ii) the systematicity of the behaviour
> which grounds thought ascription. (p. 205)

And he says (1991):

> (iii) What stands in need of computational explanation is not
> the systematicity of *thought* per se, but (iv) the systematicity of
> the behaviour which holistically warrants the ascription of the
> thoughts. (p. 215)

The inserted numerals are mine. I will first comment on conjuncts
(ii) and (iv), and then on conjuncts (i) and (ii).

To begin, I agree with (ii); Clark is certainly right that 'the systematicity of the behaviour which grounds thought ascription is in
need of empirical explanation'. The behaviour of which Clark
speaks is non-intentional overt bodily behaviour and dispositions
to behave overtly of the sort we ordinarily take as evidence for
thought-ascriptions. As I understand systematicity, behavioural
dispositions will be systematically related if and only if they have
constitutive bases such that a typical possessor of the one would
possess the other. Systematic relationships among behavioural dispositions would impose a constraint on any functional analyses of
such dispositions, namely that the analyses describe constitutive
bases for the dispositions that explain why a typical possessor of
one would possess the other. We expect neuroscience to yield
functional analyses of such non-intentional behaviourial dispositions and capacities.

Turn to claim (iv), the claim that 'the systematicity of the behaviour which holistically warrants the ascription of the thoughts stands
in need of *computational* explanation' (emphasis mine). This is a con-
tentious claim about the kind of empirical theory of non-intentional
behaviour that we should seek. It is, I think, an open question
whether such behaviour requires a *computational* explanation.

In any case, let us turn to Clark's claims (i) and (iii). To begin, I
have agreed for the sake of argument, you will recall, that generalizations of type (CG) are conceptual truths. I take it that that is
essentially what Clark means when he says that it is a conceptual
truth that thought is ceteris paribus systematic. Given that, I am
prepared to agree (for the sake of argument), that 'the systematicity of thought is not need of empirical explanation' and that 'the
systematicity of thought per se is not in need of computational
explanation.' Indeed, a stronger claim is warranted: *it makes no*

sense to speak of an empirical theory (whether a computational theory or not) explaining systematicity. For it makes no sense to speak of an empirical theory explaining generalizations of type (CG), if such generalizations are indeed conceptual truths.

None the less, Fodor's and Pylyshyn's condition of adequacy could be easily recast in a way that is consistent with generalizations of type (CG) being conceptual truths. For a theory of cognition must still satisfy (CA): it must describe constitutive bases for capacities to have intentional states. And given that, if truths of the form (CG) are conceptual truths, then they impose an *a priori* condition of adequacy on any functional analyses of the capacities in question. It would be *a priori* true that constitutive bases for such capacities are such that it is at least nomologically impossible for an individual to possess a base for one such capacity and to lack a base for the other, and yet be typical possessor of the first capacity. For a constitutive base for a capacity to have an intentional state will be a condition that is at least nomologically sufficient for possession of the capacity. Thus, if it were nomologically possible for a typical possessor of one member of a relevant pair of capacities to fail to possess a base for the other member, then it would be nomologically possible for a typical possessor of the first member to fail to possess the second. But that would imply the denial of our assumption that it is a conceptual truth that a typical possessor of the first would have the second. For given that assumption, it is nomologically impossible for a typical possessor of one member of a relevant pair to fail to possess a base for the other member of the relevant pair.[22]

Suppose, then, that generalizations of type (CG) are indeed conceptual truths. Then, the Fodor–Pylyshyn condition of adequacy can be recast as follows: to be an adequate theory of cognition, the constitutive bases the theory postulates for the members of a pair of capacities alike in ways (I) and (II) should be such that it is at least nomologically impossible for a typical possessor of one of the

---

[22] Compare the fact that it is (arguably) a conceptual truth that, ceteris paribus, water-soluble things would dissolve were they placed in water. Given that, any proposed constitutive basis of water-solubility had better be such that something with that basis would dissolve were it placed in water (under the relevant boundary conditions); otherwise, it would be *nomologically* possible for a water-soluble thing to fail to be such that it would dissolve were it placed in water under the relevant boundary conditions. And it is, by hypothesis, *conceptually* impossible for a water-soluble thing to fail to be such that it would dissolve were it placed in water (under the relevant boundary conditions). (Whatever is conceptually impossible is, of course, *ipso facto* nomologically impossible.)

capacities to have the one constitutive base but not the other. And the condition of adequacy would be an *a priori* condition of adequacy on any theory that purports to offer functional analyses of capacities to have intentional states. The Fodor–Pylyshyn challenge to connectionists would be to say how connectionism could meet this *a priori* condition of adequacy without implementing a classical cognitive architecture.

Some closing remarks about Clark's position are in order. Clark seems to be claiming that connectionism is concerned to offer an empirical theory, indeed a computational theory, of non-intentional behaviour and behavioural dispositions and capacities.[23] He seems to be denying that connectionism is concerned to offer functional analyses of capacities to have intentional states (or to engage in intentional activities); connectionism, as he characterizes it, is concerned to offer functional analyses of non-intentional dispositions and capacities to behave.[24] If Clark is right that connectionism is not concerned to offer functional analyses of capacities to have intentional states, then connectionism is not in competition with classicism. For classicism seeks to offer such functional analyses. Moreover, connectionism would not, then, have to concern itself with explaining systematicity. For the issue of explaining systematicity arises only for a theory that seeks to offer such functional analyses.

I should note, finally, that I think Clark is flatly wrong in his characterization of the connectionist enterprise. Many connection-

[23] In so far as intentional phenomena are concerned, Clark seems at times content to point out, simply, that there are kinds of behaviour that we ordinarily take as warranting ascriptions of intentional states (and activities). (But see footnote 24 below.) We should keep in mind that possession of a capacity to have an intentional state does *not* consist in the possession of a (nonintentional) capacity to engage certain sorts of overt behaviour. And let us not confuse behaviour we take to warrant thought-ascriptions with constitutive bases for the thoughts so ascribed. (I am not suggesting that Clark is guilty of this confusion.)

[24] There is, however, an independent theme in Clark (1991) that he does not separate from the behaviourist theme. He applauds Smolensky's idea that there are context-dependent representations that connectionism can invoke in its explanations. Here are two points in response: First, Smolensky (1991) proposes that we appeal to context-dependent representations in offering (what I have called following Cummins) functional analyses of intentional capacities; Smolensky is not concerned with 'the behaviour that warrants thought ascriptions'. Second, connectionism will not be able to explain systematic relationships among capacities to have intentional states by invoking context-dependent representations. For a detailed discussion of why, see Fodor and McLaughlin (1990).

ists *are* concerned to provide functional analyses of capacities to have intentional states (see, e.g., Rumelhart and McClelland 1986). Many connectionists seek to tell us what possession of capacities to have intentional states consists in, to offer constitutive bases for such capacities. It is to these connectionists that Fodor and Pylyshyn pose their challenge.

7. Can Systematicity be Explained Selectively?

Braddon-Mitchell and Fitzpatrick (1990) and Sterelny (1990) bill themselves as holding that systematic relationships amongst cognitive capacities are empirical facts to be explained. But they deny that such facts must be explained by a theory of cognition, and so they reject Fodor's and Pylyshyn's adequacy condition.

Using 'LOT' as an acronym for Language of Thought Architecture, and speaking of 'the capacities of systematicity and productivity', Braddon-Mitchell and Fitzpatrick (1989) claim that:

> the presence of these capacities can be adequately explained without the postulation of some specific mechanism or state of an organism which neatly and elegantly captures features of the organism which are visible at the behavioural level. Such an explanation is to be had from, roughly, the pressure of evolutionary forces. An evolutionary style of explanation raises the probability that a cognitive system generates systematicity and productivity without the commitment to a specific mechanism such as the LOT. (p.15)

Citing their view with approval, Sterelny (1990) remarks:

> It is easy to slide from the claim that systematicity is a functional, rather than an implementational, feature of our mental life to the idea that it is to be explained by the basic architecture of our cognitive system. But that is a slide that can be resisted, as Braddon-Mitchell and Fitzpatrick point out. They agree that it is a functional fact that mental representation is not punctuate. But they offer a diachronic rather than a synchronic explanation. Punctuate mental lives are bad for your reproductive prospects. For a punctuate mind is incapable of having some thoughts, including, perhaps, survival and reproduction enhancing ones. So natural selection will tend to build a non-punctuate mind. Minds are typically systematic. That is no accident, but the explanation is selective rather than architectural. A connectionist does not have to believe that the systematicity of intelligence is a change byproduct, an idiosyncracy. (p. 182)

Systematicity, Conceptual Truth, and Evolution

I am uncertain what Sterelny means by 'a punctate mind' or by saying that 'systematicity is a functional, rather than an implementation, feature of our mental life.' But rather than pursuing such matters, let us consider whether an appeal to natural selection can enable a cognitive theory to skirt the task of explaining systematicity.

To begin, let us concede, for the sake of argument, Braddon-Mitchell's, Fitzpatrick's, and Sterelny's tacit assumption that phenotypes are units of natural selection. Granting phenotypes are units of selection, it is straightforward that pairs of phenotypes can be co-adaptive. The shape and colour of stick insects, for example, are co-adaptive: given their shape and colour they appear to be a twigs, thereby eluding predators. And as a result these traits were co-adapted. Capacities to have intentional states are phenotypes. Let us grant that capacities alike in ways (I) and (II) are phenotypic traits that are co-adaptive and, as a result, were selected for.[25]

Natural selection could offer one sort of explanation of why capacities alike in ways (I) and (II) are highly statistically correlated: it is no accident that they are highly statistically correlated since the capacities are co-adaptive and, as a result, were selected for. Natural selection could even offer one sort of explanation of why a statistically average possessor of today, so to speak, of one member of a relevant pair of capacities would possess the other. I suspect that Braddon-Mitchell and Fitzpatrick and Sterelny may have thought that this would count as explaining systematicity. I suspect that they may have mistakenly thought that in claiming that systematically related cognitive capacities are 'intrinsically connected' rather than 'punctate', Fodor and Pylyshyn just meant (roughly) that the capacities tend to be co-possessed. Otherwise, it is hard to see how Braddon-Mitchell *et al.* could have thought that natural selection could help to explain systematicity.

But, in any case, appeals to natural selection will not, of course, tell us what the constitutive bases are for capacities to have intentional states. Thus, such appeals won't explain systematicity. For to explain systematicity, one must, you will recall, describe constitutive bases for members of relevant pairs of capacities that yield an explanation of why a typical possessor of one member of such a

[25] As Christopher Hookway mentioned to me, that is pretty implausible were many pairs of capacities alike in ways (I) and (II) are concerned: consider the capacity to believe that the electron attracted the proton and the capacity to believe that the proton attracted the electron. Quite. Surely, what were selected for are more fundamental capacities possession of which constitute possession of these capacities. And the task for a functional analysis of such capacities is, of course, to describe the more fundamental capacities in question.

pair would possess the other. It is a condition of adequacy on a cognitive theory that it say what possession of capacities to have intentional states consists in. Selective explanations won't tell us that. It is also the case that a typical possessor of one member of a relevant pair of capacities would possess the other. And it is a condition of adequacy on an account of the constitutive bases of capacities to have intentional states that the account describe constitutive bases for members of such pairs that explain why a typical possessor of one member would have the other. A selective explanation will not meet this condition of adequacy.

Now it is, of course, open to a connectionist to respond by denying that capacities alike in ways (I) and (II) have constitutive bases such that a typical possessor of the one would have the other. This would be to deny that the capacities are systematically related. But it is open to a connectionist to deny that. The connectionist could deny it and yet still maintain that capacities alike in ways (I) and (II) are highly, and non-accidentally, statistically correlated.

A connectionist who took this line would, of course, have to disagree with Clark about whether counterfactual generalizations of type (CG) are conceptual truths. For if they are conceptual truths, then a functional analysis of the members of a relevant pair of capacities would have to ascribe to them constitutive bases such that it is nomologically impossible for an individual to possess one base and not the other, and yet be a typical possessor of the one relevant cognitive capacity. But in denying that counterfactual generalizations of type (CG) are conceptual truths, such connectionist would not, of course, be disagreeing with Fodor and Pylyshyn; for Fodor and Pylyshyn deny that the generalizations are conceptual truths. However, notice also that a connectionist who took the line in question would have to deny that the possession of capacities of the sorts cited in (1)–(4) consist of the possession of the same concepts and a faculty for exercising the concepts in either of the two ways in question. For if they conceded that point, then the capacities would be systematically related. The challenge to connectionists, then, would be to explain what possession of the concepts and of the faculty consist in without appeal to an architecture that implements a classical architecture.

But suppose the connectionist denied that the capacities cited in (1)–(4) are systematically related. That position may well, contra Clark, be a logically coherent; but it seems to me wildly implausible. A proper defense of the claim that capacities like those cited in (1)–(4) are systematically related is beyond the scope of this essay. But it should be mentioned that possession of the members of the pairs in question certainly consist, in part, in possession of the capacity to be in states in the relevant intentional modes. For example, both possession of the capacity to believe *that the cat is chasing the dog* and of the capacity to believe *that the dog is chasing the cat* consists, in part, in possession of the capacity to have beliefs. Moreover, given the contents of the two beliefs, it seems quite implausible that the two capacities lack constitutive bases that explain why a possessor of a capacity to have the one belief would also possess the capacity to have the other. Finally, Braddon-Mitchell and Fitzpatrick and Sterelny give us no reason at all to doubt that capacities alike in ways (I) and (II) have constitutive bases such that a typical possessor of the one would possess the other.

If such capacities are so related, that imposes a condition of adequacy on any theory that purports to offer functional analyses of the capacities, namely that it offer functional analyses of the capacities that yield an explanation of why a typical possessor of one would possess the other. Given this condition of adequacy, if connectionism seeks to offer functional analyses of capacities to have intentional states, then connectionists face the Fodor-Pylyshyn challenge: to tell us how connectionism proposes to do this without proposing an architecture that implements a classical cognitive architecture. Appeals to natural selection will not enable connectionists to skirt this challenge. And if it is a conceptual truth that capacities alike in ways (I) and (II) are systematically related, the Fodor-Pylyshyn challenge can, as we saw, be easily recast; indeed it can be recast in a way that makes it even more formidable.

References

Block, N. 1982. *Imagery*. Cambridge, MA: MIT Press.

Braddon-Mitchell, D. & Fitzpatrick, J. 1990. Explanation and the language of thought. *Synthese*, **83**, 3–29.

Clark, A. 1988. Thoughts, sentences and cognitive science. *Philosophical Psychology*, **1**, 263–278.

Clark, A. 1989. *Microcognition*. Cambridge MA: MIT/Bradford.

Clark, A. 1991. Systematicity structured representations and cognitive architecture: a reply to Fodor and Pylyshyn. In Horgan and Tienson 1991, pp. 198–218.

Crane, T. (ed.) 1992a. *The Contents of Experience: Essays on Perception*. Cambridge: Cambridge University Press.

Crane, T. 1992b. The nonconceptual content of experience. In Crane 1992a, pp. 136–137.

Cummins, R. 1983. *The Nature of Psychological Explanation*. Cambridge MA: MIT/Bradford.

Davies, M. 1991. Concepts, connectionism, and the language of thought. In Ramsey, *et al*, pp. 229–258.

Dennett, D. 1991. Mother nature versus the walking encyclopedia: a western drama. In Ramsey *et al.* 1991, pp. 21–30.

Dretske, F. 1978. The role of the percept in visual cognition. In C. Wade Savage (ed.) *Perception and Cognition: Issues in the Foundations of Psychology, Minnesota Studies in the Philosophy of Science*, Vol. IX. Minneapolis: University of Minnesota Press, pp. 107–128.

Dretske, F. 1991. *Explaining Behaviour: Reasons in a World of Causes.* Cambridge MIT/Bradford Book.

Evans, G. 1982. *Varieties of Reference.* Oxford: Oxford University Press.

Fodor, J. 1975. *The Language of Thought.* New York: Thomas Crowell, and Cambridge Mass: Harvard University Press.

Fodor, J. 1982. Imagistic representation. In Block 1982, pp. 63–86.

Fodor, J. & Pylyshyn, Z. 1988. Connectionism and cognitive architecture: a critical analysis. *Cognition,* **28,** 3–71.

Fodor, J. (1990). *A Theory of Content and Other Essays.* Cambridge MA: MIT/Bradford.

Fodor, J. & McLaughlin, B. P. 1990. Connectionism and the problem of systematicity: why Smolensky's solution doesn't work. *Cognition,* **35,** 183–204.

Goldman, A. 1986. *Epistemology and Cognition.* Cambridge: Harvard University Press.

Heil, J. 1989. *Cause, Mind, and Reality.* Kluwer.

Horgan, T. & Tienson, J. 1991. *Connectionism and the Philosophy of Mind .* Kluwer.

Loewer, B. & Rey, G. 1991. *Meaning in Mind.* Oxford: Basil Blackwell.

Matthews, R. 1991. Is there vindication through representationalism? In Loewer & Rey 1991, pp. 137–150.

McLaughlin, B. P. 1987. Tye on connectionism. *Spindel Conference on Connectionism, Southern Journal of Philosophy,* **26,** 185–193.

McLaughlin, B. P. 1989. Why perception is not singular reference. In Heil 1989, pp. 111–120.

McLaughlin, B. P. 1993a. On punctate content and on conceptual role. *Philosophy and Phenomenological Research,* **3,** 653–660.

McLaughlin, B. P. 1993b. The classicism/connectionism battle to win souls. *Philosophical Studies,* **70,** 45–72.

McLaughlin, B. P. & Warfield, T. A. Forthcoming. The allures of connectionism reexamined. *Synthese.*

Peacocke, C. 1992. Scenarios, concepts and perception. In Crane 1992a, pp. 105–135.

Ramsey, W., Stich, S. P. & Rumelhart, D. E. 1991. *Philosophy and Connectionist Theory.* Hillsdale: Erlbaum.

Rumelhart, D. E. & McClelland, J. L. 1986. *Parallel Distributed Processing,* Cambridge MA: MIT Press.

Schiffer, S. 1991. Does mentalese have a compositional semantics? In Loewer & Rey 1991, pp. 181–200.

Smolensky, 1991. Connectionism, constituency and the language of thought. In Loewer & Rey, pp. 201–228.

Sterelny, K. 1990. *The Representational Theory of the Mind.* Oxford: Basil Blackwell.

Tye, M. 1992. Visual qualia and visual content. In Crane 1992a, pp. 158–176.

Index of Names

[Names mentioned in footnotes and in parentheses are not included.]

Index of Names

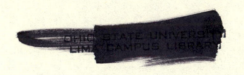